MAKE
FOOD
SIMPLE

TAKE STRESS AND CONFUSION OUT OF
NUTRITION AND MAKE QUICK, HEALTHY
MEALS FOR THE ENTIRE FAMILY

DR. LIVINGOOD
JESSICA LIVINGOOD

GRAPHICS & EDITING BY
MORGAN FERGUSON

MAKE FOOD SIMPLE
By Dr. Livingood and Jessica Livingood

1st Printing, May 2019
Printed in the United States of America

DEDICATION

TO ANYONE STRUGGLING TO
EXPERIENCE REAL HEALTH.
MAKE FOOD SIMPLE.

TABLE OF CONTENTS

CHAPTER 1   9
THE WAR AGAINST CHRONIC
DISEASE

CHAPTER 2   17
THE PLAN

CHAPTER 3   25
CUT THE SUGAR

CHAPTER 4   31
CRANK UP GOOD FAT

CHAPTER 5   41
CLEAN UP THE TOXINS

CHAPTER 6   61
CARE ABOUT NUTRIENTS &
CURB CONSUMPTION

LETTER FROM JESSICA   73
LIVINGOOD

LETTER FROM DR. LIVINGOOD   74

PANTRY LIST   76

FAMILIES & LITTLES   78

EVERY DAY FOOD LIST   80

ANTI-INFLAMMATORY FOOD LIST   82

RECIPES   85

THE WAR AGAINST CHRONIC DISEASE

Procrastination is the thief of health.

Is there something you know you should be doing with your health right now and you are simply not doing it? You see, we get it. As Americans, we understand that the choices we make every single day are not leading to a lifetime of experiencing real health. 75% of Americans, in fact, believe that obesity is caused by lifestyle, not disease. Almost half of Americans believe that fast food is bad for them, 67% of U.S. adults believe that public school lunches should meet standards for nutritional values, and one out of four American teens are seriously trying to lose weight. We get it.

Yet we don't get it. In the United States, 63.1% of American adults are now overweight and a whopping--no pun intended--35.7% are obese. Heart disease deaths in the United States occur once every 34 seconds. That's 1,726 heart disease deaths a day. Every day, cancer in the United States is claiming over 1,500 lives, and 3,400 people get the dreaded diagnosis.

We get it. We understand that our lifestyle is leading to our own demise, but we don't "get it" because we're refusing to act and procrastinating when it comes to our health. None of us actually believe it will happen to us. America right now is by far the most obese nation in the world. Almost 36% of our entire country of men, women, and children are obese. (Out of the top 30 countries in the world, Japan ranks the best at 3.5%. We are 10 times larger than Japan.) Despite our spending the most on healthcare per capita in the world, obesity is taking its toll on our country and its culture.

There's no profit in teaching people to walk or exercise more. There's no profit in teaching people to breathe, relax, and de-stress from the craziness of their lives. These lifestyles are causing an epidemic of more than 150 million Americans currently affected. This equates to six in ten people living with a chronic disease. Four out of 10 of those people have two or more diseases. Chronic disease refers to heart disease, cancer, diabetes, kidney failure, lung disease, stroke or Alzheimer's. They cost our country $3.3 trillion in healthcare costs every year. Chronic diseases are very preventable diseases which drive an enormous healthcare cost and are responsible for 40% of all deaths, according to the CDC. It has become obvious that nearly all cases of chronic disease are treatable and preventable with proper diet and a proper lifestyle.

The chronic disease epidemic is fueled by the fact that we don't actually have a healthcare system. When Dennis Cortese, the former director of Mayo Clinic, was asked how he would fix our healthcare system, his response sums it up. He says, "You can't fix something that doesn't exist. It's like going out to your garage to fix your car and getting into your garage and realizing, oh, I don't have a car. You cannot fix something that doesn't exist."

In America, if you do not have a diagnosis, our healthcare system cannot help you. You literally have to be sick in order to enter what we call a healthcare system. If all you're doing is waiting around to get diagnosed with a sickness or disease, or treating and managing sickness or disease with a drug or a surgery, that's not healthcare. That's sick care. The system is not designed to get you healthy or even to get to the cause of the issue in the first place. We have the largest "sick care" system in the world. We spend more on sick care than any other country, and it shows because we're sick.

The guidelines to our healthcare run through our federal health insurance program Medicare. Whether you have Medicare or not, they are calling the shots. Now, I don't expect you to dive into the Medicare guideline book, but I think you should pay attention to Medicare because they make all the decisions to dictate what your health insurance does and doesn't do. It dictates what your doctor does or doesn't do. We typically only do what our insurance pays for, so what does it pay for? Check out section 2251.3 of the Medicare guidelines:

"A treatment plan that seeks to prevent disease, promote health, and prolong and enhance the quality of life or therapy that is performed to maintain or prevent deterioration of a chronic condition is not medically necessary."

The leading entity of all healthcare decisions and our sick care system in the United States says that things that need to be done to prevent disease or prolong your health are just not necessary. The entire system is not set up to make you healthier and lead you to a prosperous life without drugs and surgeries. There's no profit in teaching people to eat more vegetables, exercise, and de-stress.

Your health is your responsibility.
No one is coming for you.

This book is designed to equip you to take care of one of the biggest causes of disease...food. Before we fix your food, let's see where you are by listening to what your body is telling you.

Below is a list of common conditions that are fast-tracking you down the road to heart disease, lung disease, cancer, Alzheimer's, stroke, kidney failure, or becoming one of the 6 out of 10 Americans that have a chronic disease.

High Triglycerides
High Blood Pressure
High Blood Sugar
Low Blood Sugar
High Insulin
High Leptin
Toxicity
ADD/ADHD
Autism Spectrum Disorder
Inflammation or Joint Pain

Cancer
Chronic Fatigue
Thyroid Problems
Fibromyalgia
Lupus
Digestive Dysfunction
Acid Reflux/Heartburn
Obesity
Inability to Lose Weight
Gluten Sensitivities

So, where are you? Are you on the path to being one of the 6 out of 10 that has a chronic disease? Do you already have a chronic disease? Do any of your family members have a chronic disease? If so, what choices are you making that are causing the problem? What do you know you need to do better when it comes to your health?

You don't get to sit back and blame genetics. In fact, Time magazine says that 98% of disease is not due to the genes you are given. It's due to the choices you make every single day. It's due to your lifestyle--and 100% of disease can be impacted and improved by your lifestyle. Maybe not reversed, maybe not completely cured--but every disease and every condition can be improved when you take better care of yourself. Essentially what I'm saying is that if you can "lifestyle" your way into it, you can "lifestyle" your way out of it.

If you are dealing with any of the above conditions, research is now very clear that you can do something about it. Your lifestyle can be changed and these conditions can be improved, and, as I've seen thousands of times, completely reversed. You just have to start making the right choices. This book was written because the biggest reason that we're dealing with so much chronic disease in this country is (because of) what is and isn't going into our mouths.

WE ARE WHAT WE EAT

Of an average grocery budget, 23% goes to processed foods, bagged chips, bagged crackers, and sweets, 22% goes to meat, 15% to grains and baked goods, while only 15% is left over for green leafy vegetables and healthy wholesome foods. The primary food that we're eating is made up of sugars (grains) and processed foods.

We are what we eat. Statistics show that 48% of Americans drink a soda at least once a day and 70% of our caloric intake is from processed foods. More than seven out of ten foods that we put into our bodies are processed, man-made, and foreign. Our body does not know what to do with it. Only 59% of our meals served at home are homemade. A whopping 80% of popular US food today contains ingredients that are actually banned in other countries.

No wonder we're number one on the list of industrialized nations in years of potential life lost. No wonder we're number one on the list of the amount of chronic disease. No wonder we're spending the most money on sick care than anyone else in the world.

> We have disease from excess food while other countries have disease from too little.

So what's the barrier? Do you know there is something you need to be doing with your health right now and you are simply not doing it? Do you know you need to eat better and simply do not? Procrastination is the thief of health. You don't need to be perfect; you just need to begin. If you know you need to improve your nutrition.....If we know and we "get it" and we realize the choices we make are driving us to have a chronic disease at the rate of 6 out of 10 Americans, then what are the barriers that are holding us back from making the right choices? If we can break through these barriers, we can finally experience real health.

...The battle is between the ears. The battle is underneath your quarter-inch skull. You don't need more information, more handouts, or more movies--you just need knowledge. There's a big difference between knowledge and information. We're in the information age. We have more information than we've ever had. More information is not going to change your life. What will change your life is knowledge, and knowledge is the application of information. People perish without knowledge. I truly believe that if you do not apply what you are learning, it does you no good.

> Information will not change your life. What will change your life is knowledge, and knowledge is the application of information.

So the last thing I would want you to do is to read this book and then not apply it into your life and your family's life. I believe that in order to apply it, you need it to be simple. The number one thing holding you back is that there is so much conflicting information and misinformation. This book was written to help you simplify your food and simplify your health.

The second barrier is taste. It still has to taste good! You don't want to give up the feeling of good, tasty food. I get it. I love it. There are a lot of foods that aren't good for me that I still enjoy to eat, but if we can get good, nutritious, wholesome food in your body and not leave you feeling deprived, you'll succeed. Most of us are living to eat instead of eating to live. It's time you start transforming your mind from short-term crash diets and short-term weight-loss goals to long-term values. The most important thing that you're going to need in order to experience your retirement, play with your grandbabies, and serve out your purpose on the earth is your health. Act like it. Eat like it.

The third barrier is the budget: it costs too much to eat healthily. Anyone that ever says this to me has never experienced disease in this country, because you are only one diagnosis away from bankruptcy. I've lived it. My dad lost his health suddenly at age 51. He was on no drugs and had passed every physical for over 30 years. On the inside, he was unhealthy and didn't know it. I saw my dad lose his greatest asset, his health. I then had a front seat to the thing I am trying to prevent all of you from ever having to go through, and that is the American healthcare system. Trying to get healthy after you've lost your health in a sick care system is almost impossible, and it will bankrupt you.

I saw my dad put on 15 drugs, have open-heart surgery then, on January 5, 2008, lose his hearing. He couldn't bike, couldn't work, couldn't fish, or spend time with his family. He lost his health and then lost everything, including his money. His medical debt cost our family over $200,000. It ate away at my dad's retirement, and we nearly lost it all.

You can't afford cancer. You can't afford the surgery. You can't afford to be sick. You can't afford to not be able to work. You can't afford to not be able to provide for your family. Disease costs too much. Health is cheap compared to disease. It's just a matter of prioritization. Put down the fast food and stop spending so much on things that destroy your body. Focus on buying quality nutrients and food to fuel the most important vehicle you have, your body.

Finally, maybe you've tried and failed. You've tried so many different diets, so many different approaches, and most of them are unsustainable. So the purpose of this book is to un-diet. Not to crash you down to lower weights or get short-term results that make you look good for a few weeks. Not to ignore the type of eating that as soon as you stop doing it, you immediately go back to where you began.

I failed with my father for years. It is because I failed that this book exists. Failure brings success. We learn when we fail. Health is arguably the most valuable thing you have. You have to fight for it! If there is one thing to never stop pursuing, it is your health. You have to have it to live out your purpose and life. The following chapters are part of the plan that got my dad his life back. After years of failure, we learned how to experience real health, and the core was making food simple.

It's time for you to break through those past failures of dieting and for you to finally learn how to experience real health by making food simple. I truly believe that straight from our kitchen to yours and straight from our family to yours, you now hold the tool that can make eating fun and delicious while it builds health and protects the most important asset you have--you! However, procrastination is the thief of health. So it's time to begin!

2

THE PLAN

Eat to live don't live to eat.

There are two approaches in this book. One gets you to your health goals as fast as possible while the second helps you stay there for a lifetime. The Plan gets you experiencing real health--not treating a condition, not relying on a drug for the rest of your life, not losing 15 pounds and then a couple of months later putting it back on, but actually keeping you healthy. Hitting the goal is easy; keeping the goal is the challenging part.

THE CHALLENGE PLAN

In the last chapter, we discussed a whole list of different symptoms. If you have those symptoms and you're facing those diseases and conditions that are going to lead you to chronic disease, then it's time to buckle down. It's time to take the challenge, and it's time to get serious about your nutrition.

If you need hormone repair...
If your weight loss (or gain) is out of control...
If you are on prescription drugs...
If you're resistant to sugar...
If you've turned into a sugar burner or carb addict...
If you have extra weight on your waistline...
If you are a sugar burner or carb addict and need to gain weight...
If you have a lot of inflammation...
If your gut is breaking down or inflamed...
If your joints are sore and hurting...
If you have intolerances to food...

If you need accelerated weight loss to get the weight off quickly and the tools to keep it off...

If it's just time for a complete health restoration because you're dealing with blood pressure, blood sugar, triglyceride problems or any of the many other common related issues that cause metabolic conditions, then...

It's time to take the challenge. It's time to make food simple through the Challenge Plan.

THE EVERDAY PLAN

If you've reached your health goals then the harder part is staying that way. The quicker we can get you to your health goals is goal number one. Goal two is to keep you on a plan that you can do every day, yet still cheat occasionally, and maintain your results forever. This is the Everyday Plan. The Everyday Plan is the nutritional plan that my family uses day in day out to raise three healthy kids and keep my wife and myself healthy, energized, serving our purpose and full of energy and life.

If God made it, eat it. If He didn't, don't.

The focus is real food, not a diet, not restriction, not calories, but real food. If God made it, eat it. If He didn't, don't. It's a pretty easy principle to live by. Whatever your beliefs are, eating real food just works. Most diets, if you are on one, will still work under this plan because every diet incorporates real food. If it does not, then you may want to rethink your approach. Nothing beats real food. Calorie counting and restriction may even work on this plan, but instead of counting calories, start counting nutrients because if your body gets enough nutrients, it will work the way it's designed to.

VACATION MEALS

This will be your favorite part. The Everyday Plan gives you the freedom to be human. Go ahead and mess up. Just don't do it every day. I call them vacation meals. You can call them your vices. Just enjoy whatever it is you want to enjoy. An Oreo cookie, a piece of pizza, beer, whatever it is, go for it. Just don't do it daily. How often do you go on vacation--four to twelve times per year? Then that's how often you can have a total cheat day of a certain food. The everyday plan is to build health every day, not eat junk food every day. You can have and enjoy different foods while you're on vacation and then when you come back from vacation, get back on track.

The problem is many are on vacation
(...Every. Single. Day.)

Are you always treating yourself in little ways and have an emotional addiction to food? If you can cut this out with the Challenge Plan, breaking the addictions and habits as we'll show you to do, then you'll get a greater appreciation for real food. You'll curb your taste buds back to wanting and craving real food as opposed to the sugary processed mess that man has created.

Break your addiction, occasionally enjoy bad food, and live normally. That's the Everyday Plan. You can still have a birthday treat. You can still have a holiday meal. Just do it within reason and respond with healthy eating and habits afterward. If you get off track, don't beat yourself up. Just respond. If you enjoy a little bit too much or have a weak moment, just respond. The Everyday Plan sets you up to know how to eat real food to get back on track when the vacation days throw you off.

THE HEALING POWER OF MAKING FOOD SIMPLE

The purpose of the (make food simple book) is fourfold. I believe if you can get these four things under control, you can get to the root cause of hundreds of conditions that now face our society.

1. BURN FAT

How can you turn yourself into a fat-burning machine? How do you burn fat for fuel instead of sugar? The best analogy is to think of it as fuel for your car.

If your car runs off unleaded fuel, you can't put diesel in and expect it to work very well. The same applies to your body. If you want to be a fat burner, you can't put sugar in. We'll refer to sugar as diesel. It burns unclean, it slows you down, and it adds on a bunch of extra weight. Fat is unleaded fuel. Actually, it's more like rocket fuel. Fat burns much more cleanly and leaves less soot and damage behind once it burns. If you want to burn fat, you have to fuel your body with fat. Fuel your vehicle with what you want it to burn. The fuel is up to you. Everything that goes in is either going to burn fat or store fat. It's as simple as that.

Fat Burners rely on fat for energy. They burn fat in their sleep. They extract more energy from less food. For fat burners, fat is the preferred fuel source inside their body, and they will lose weight on any diet.

Sugar burners rely on sugar for energy. They've forgotten how to burn fat. Their metabolism is shot. They require regular sugar for energy. Sound familiar? Therefore sugar burners have uncontrollable cravings for their fuel. They also plateau on a diet and can't get any lower or lose weight at all.

Sugar burners require the Challenge to reset the system, reset the metabolism, and turn the fat burning machine back on.

2. DETOX

The second purpose of the Make Food Simple plan is to fix your filters.

We live in a toxic society. There are over 3,000 chemicals used in the storage and processing of our food. Over 10,000 chemicals are used in all of the food supply, and over 70,000 chemicals used in the processing of materials, building supplies, and all other industries.

Here is the best way you can determine if you're toxic right now. You don't need a test. You don't need a doctor or some special diagnosis. If you have a pulse inside of your body, then rest assured you're toxic. If you're reading this book right now, you're toxic. We all need to address it, and God gave you some amazing filtration systems to deal with this issue--Your liver, kidneys, digestive tract, skin, lymph system, and fat cells. It's as if He knew you were going to get bombarded. If you can regularly help those filters out, you can allow your body to work the way it's supposed to.

You are made of 17 trillion cells. Healthy cells=healthy you. If your cells can get good in and bad out, you're going to be healthy. If your cells get congested and toxic, good things can't get into the cells and bad things can't get out of the cells. Cellular congestion leaves you in a toxic state. Toxic cells are the cause of metabolic conditions like heart disease, cancer, and failed organs. The second goal of the Make Food Simple plan is to detox your body by changing what you eat to crank up the filters inside of your body. Stop toxifying yourself by eating right so your filters can remove the toxins.

3. REDUCE INFLAMMATION: SEVERAL YEARS BACK IN TIME

magazine's cover story called inflammation the secret killer and highlighted its surprising link with heart attacks, cancer, Alzheimer's and other chronic diseases.

The root of almost every chronic disease is this self-inflicted burning damage. External damage can certainly harm you. You can damage yourself by falling, by overly-repetitive use of your hands (such as typing on a keyboard causing carpal tunnel syndrome) or by wearing out your knees by being too hard on them over the years. Internal damage caused by food is worse.

Excess sugar and toxic food end up in your bloodstream and damage your blood vessels from the inside out. It scars your tissue, slows your organs, and tears up the inside of your body. The body then responds with inflammation. The inflammation shows up to attempt to heal the damage. The damage just keeps coming like a never-ending storm.

A storm of fast food, diet sodas, overeating, disrupting

toxins, and chemical destroyers found in food. The body calls in more first responders, inflammation, to weather the storm to attempt to protect the body. Over time the system weakens from the inflammation and begins to break down. The inflammation shuts down organs like a bad storm shuts down businesses. The inflammation shuts down the heart. It shuts down the liver. It backs up sugar which results in diabetes and leads to cellular destruction like cancer. Bad food fuels the storm, and fixing it extinguishes the inflammation.

4. BALANCE YOUR HORMONES

The primary hormones that the Make Food Simple plan is focused on are insulin and leptin. They apply to men and women alike. These hormones are your sugar-burning hormone and your fat-burning hormone respectively. If your diet primarily consists of carbohydrates and the incredible amount of sugar that most of us eat in a day, then insulin, your sugar-storage hormone, goes higher and higher. (The higher insulin is required to respond the more burnt out it gets.) It stops working, and the carbs and excess energy are stored as fat.

The storage of fat from the insulin burnout increases leptin. Leptin is made by fat, and its job is to shut down your appetite so that you stop eating. With so much insulin and so much fat storage, your body becomes resistant to leptin and stops hearing the message, hence the constant cravings and addiction to food. Think about it--a person that has 20 to 40 extra pounds of fat should have no reason to be hungry. There should be plenty of excess energy to burn off before needing to eat.

Your hormones should work like a thermostat,always resetting back down to the comfortable,ideal temperature. Insulin is like cold air, and leptin is like hot air. When the body's thermostat stops sensing what insulin is telling it, then it starts storing fat. The fat-burning furnace starts getting cold. The body Insulin goes up, and the body gains fat and increases leptin; but when leptin breaks and the body becomes resistant to it, there's nothing to shut off that appetite. So we eat and we eat and we eat. And this is how fast food chains like Taco Bell exploit our broken leptin, our broken metabolisms, and allow us to eat late until 2:00 AM and continue to feed the broken system.

Does your metabolism thermostat need a reset? Do you need to turn the heat up on your fat-burning furnace? We need to reset and shock the system to repair the insulin resistance and repair the leptin so your body can start to hear the hormone communication again.

Conquering these four key principles, I truly believe, is the solution to controlling or eliminating chronic disease. If we can get you into the fat-burning mode, remove the toxicity, reduce inflammation, and balance out your hormones, your life will change. Making food simple can do all this and break your addiction to the food you thought you loved. There's a better path. You're going to love the new way. It's the road to experiencing real health. Real health tastes sweeter than any food.

3

CUT THE SUGAR

Making food simple comes down to five main parts. I call them the five C's. I wanted to make it nice and cute for you so you could always remember them.

1. Cut the sugar.

2. Crank up good fat.

3. Clean up the toxins.

4. Care about nutrients.

5. Curb your consumption.

Let's take a look at the number one most toxic food known to Americans, sugar.

In 1700 the average person consumed about four pounds of sugar per year.

In 1800 the average person consumed 18 pounds of sugar per year.

By 1900 it rose to 90 pounds of sugar per year.

By 2009 more than 50% of all Americans consumed one half a pound of sugar per day. The Department of Health and Human Services says that every American consumes 152 pounds of sugar every year. Sixty-three pounds of it comes from high fructose corn syrup. We're on a sugar high.

Here are just a few reasons why our sugar addiction is such a big problem. Sugar is the primary dietary cause of obesity. It increases acidity in the body, which promotes disease. Sugar causes inflammation and serves as the primary source of gasoline to fuel that fire. It's the primary reason for high cholesterol and high triglycerides, as it turns to fat in the liver. It causes hormonal and metabolic imbalances, which means it breaks your metabolism. Sugar puts you on the fast track for diabetes. In the South where I live, diabetes is literally referred to as "The Sugar." It's a known toxin. Sugar leads to heart disease by damaging the blood vessels. It's an anti-nutrient, meaning not only does it have no nutritional value, but it blocks the value of real nutrients.

Sugar causes cancer. The PET scan, used to identify cancer, is a test run by injecting a sugary liquid into your arm and waiting for 30 minutes before performing the scan. The sugar molecules have radioactive dyes attached. Cancer eats the sugar, and when the scan radiates you, it can identify cancer. Cancer cells eat eight times more sugar than normal cells. Certainly not every single type of cancer, but a majority of cancers, live off of one main substance, which is sugar.

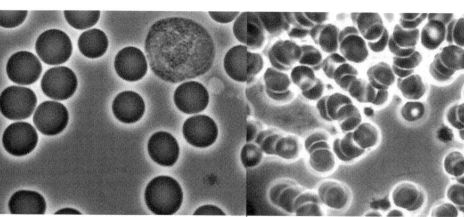

HEALTHY CELLS UNDER MICROSCOPE | 15 MINUTES AFTER 200MG OF SUGAR

If that didn't give you enough reason to break free from it, then the scariness of the addiction to it should. Substances like sugar, alcohol, and drugs release dopamine in your brain. That's your temporary happy button, which is what makes them addictive. While sugar, stimulants like alcohol and caffeine, and narcotics like cocaine initially increased dopamine release, their chronic consumption eventually causes a dopamine deficiency. This leads to a more serious anxiousness and a craving that requires a larger and larger amount of the stimulant to get the exact same effect. This addiction has been shown to be more powerful with sugar than with cocaine. I believe both should just be avoided.

The fact that sugar is a more addictive substance than cocaine has put us in a very bad spot as a country. When your body doesn't burn fat, it requires sugar for energy. At that point, your brain has two choices. It burns up its own muscle supply to supply the sugar and feed the addiction, or it gives you uncontrollable cravings that you have to listen to. If you are experiencing this, you're in sugar-burning mode.

Yet every day as a doctor, after taking care of 25,000+ patients, I hear the classic response from every addict, "I don't eat that much sugar; I don't have a sugar problem." Even if you're better than the average American and you only eat 100 pounds or of sugar a year, or even just 75 pounds, it's still a problem.

Part of the issue is that most people are not trying to hide their addiction. They just simply don't know what sugar is. People really think they don't eat that much. The moment any of a large list of food enters your body, it is turned into sugar. So just because it wasn't a sugar cookie or a piece of candy that went in your mouth doesn't mean it wasn't sugar. Let's just take a look at what sugar is and what sugar isn't.

First, companies hide it from you. They give sugar code names so you don't even know you are eating it. Here are 61 code names for sugar:

Agave nectar
Barbados sugar
Barley malt
Barley malt syrup
Beet sugar
Brown sugar
Buttered syrup
Cane juice
Cane juice crystals
Cane sugar
Caramel
Carob syrup
Castor sugar
Coconut palm sugar
Coconut sugar
Confectioner's sugar
Corn sweetener
Corn syrup
Corn syrup solids
Date sugar
Dehydrated cane juice
Demerara sugar
Dextrin
Dextrose
Evaporated cane juice
Free-flowing brown sugars
Fructose
Fruit juice
Fruit juice concentrate
Glucose
Glucose solids

Golden sugar
Golden syrup
Grape sugar
HFCS (high-fructose
          corn syrup)
Honey
Icing sugar
Invert sugar
Malt syrup
Maltodextrin
Maltol
Maltose
Mannose
Maple syrup
Molasses
Muscovado
Palm sugar
Panocha
Powdered sugar
Raw sugar
Refiner's syrup
Rice syrup
Saccharose
Sorghum syrup
Sucrose
Sugar (granulated)
Sweet sorghum
Syrup
Treacle
Turbinado sugar
Yellow sugar

If sugar is hidden everywhere in all of our products, then why don't we just go to sugar-free products? There are no calories. They taste good. Diabetics can drink them, and then they won't cause weight gain. What is the problem? The issue is toxicity. Aspartame and artificial sweeteners are chemicals that are used to mimic the taste of sugar. They're found in many of our processed foods, and they have known excitotoxins. Excitotoxins cause the neurons in your brain to excite themselves to death.

Evidence suggests that these chemicals promote cancer growth and have the increased propensity to cause it to spread. Aspartame itself causes the brain to be hypoglycemic, which can lead to brain damage, increase the risk of dementia, and cause headaches. Artificial sweeteners weaken the immune system, which increases viral infections. They have also been linked to seizures, episodic incidents of violence, learning disorders, and degenerative brain disorders.

The primary reason people choose a "diet" product is to remove sugar to maintain weight. However, research shows "diet" eaters actually gain more weight long-term because the toxins increase cravings and promote overeating.

None of these toxins are pulled from the market, and they just keep being advertised to you as a great alternative and even as "health foods". Splenda, a popular artificial sweetener, promotes that it's simply "Made from Sugar". That couldn't be further from the truth. I was a biochemistry minor in college, and I'll spare you the boring biochemistry lesson here; however, the process of making Splenda starts with sucrose, which is a form of sugar, but it takes about 14 chemical reactions and additives to get it to what we call Splenda. Its real name is 1,6-Dichloro-1,6-dideoxy-β-D-fructofuranosyl-4-chloro-4-doxy-α-D-galactopyranoside. All that means for you is that it is toxic and even more deadly.

HEALTHY SUGAR ALTERNATIVES

What are the alternatives to sugar to satisfy that sweet tooth? Again, let's just go back to our basic premise. If God made it, eat it; if He didn't, don't. Real food is the focus. We look first at plants, and one of the best is Stevia. This sweet leaf can be ground down into a sweet and friendly powder alternative. You certainly could have some sensitivity, especially if stevia is over-processed, just like any other food on this planet, but Stevia extract powder can be a great sweetener to satisfy the sweet tooth and help you overcome the sugar addiction. Be sure there are no additives to the stevia you buy. Companies are now adding maltodextrin and dextrose (see above in the list of 61 code names for sugar) into the stevia. Organic stevia--that's the only ingredient you should be looking for.

If you are sensitive or intolerant to stevia, then another alternative is Monk fruit. Monk fruit is made from an Asian melon and has similar properties to stevia. Sugar alcohols can be good replacements as well. Erythritol and xylitol are the most common, and, ideally, you want these products to be the least processed as possible and sourced from non-genetically modified foods. For example, xylitol can be sourced from corn that is highly-genetically modified. In our toxins section, we'll get into why this is a bad idea. Look for xylitol sourced from birch instead.

The bottom line is that we're in a state of sweet misery, and the deadly effects of sugar are overwhelming. It's the one thing you've got to fix, or you'll drive yourself directly into more chronic disease. Understand that you're dealing with an addiction that is stronger than cocaine. I didn't say it was going to be easy to break, but it will be worth it.

You can break the addiction; you can make your body into a fat burner again. Learn what sugar is, what sugar isn't, and start finding things that you enjoy that don't involve taking in a mega-dose of the sugary toxin. You're well on your way to accomplishing the first "C"--cutting out sugar and turning off the sugar-burning system. Now you're ready to turn on fat-burning mode.

4

CRANK UP GOOD FAT

The second "C" of making food simple is to crank up good fat. Going back to the car analogy, if you want to be a fat burner, you've got to fuel your body with fat. If you want your car to be an unleaded burner, you can't fuel it with diesel-- you've got to put unleaded in it. Your fuel pump is the dinner table. Instead of fueling your body with toxic sugar (diesel), it's time to fill your body with rocket fuel--healthy fat.

Your body loves healthy fat; it is essential to your body. People believe the myth that fat makes you fat. Fat does not make you fat. It's the inability to burn fat that makes you fat. One of the four main purposes of the Make Food Simple plan is to reset and balance out your hormones, insulin and leptin. This balance allows your body to know what to do with sugar and to understand how to burn up fat. When these hormones are off, then fat and sugar consumption become a problem.

Healthy fats also help your body burn fat and are used all throughout your system. Fat builds cell membranes. In fact, there is a fat layer around every cell inside of your body, so if you don't have good fat, you can't produce healthy new cells. Fats absorb vitamins, cushion organs, protect you from extreme temperatures, and regulate and make up the building blocks of all the hormones inside of your body. Fat lowers inflammation levels and allows proper cellular detoxification in the body. In fact,up to 70% of your brain is made up of fat!

Notice that the second "C" is Crank up the GOOD fat. There is a reason for that. You can put fat into the body, and it can be very toxic. Rancid, foreign, unrecognizable fats inside of your system cause cellular congestion and create poor cell membranes, which leads to chronic disease. The type of fat you eat is important. This, I believe, is the biggest missing piece in America's nutrition plan today. Low carb, no sugar, no toxins, no gluten, non-GMO, and other nutrition approaches are much more well- known than the dangers and impact of bad fats.

GOOD FAT VS. BAD FAT

What is bad fat and what is good fat? Let's look at bad fat first. The core principle is that a bad fat is fat made by man, processed in a factory. These are hydrogenated and partially hydrogenated oils such as cottonseed oil, soybean oil, and vegetable oils, and they hide in foods you would consider to not be fatty foods.

Bad fats are prevalent in almost every bread, grain, crackers, cookies and boxed food in America. Trans fats are good examples of these man-made fats like margarine and synthetic butter whose chemical structures resemble plastic. Canola oil is an interesting example. There is no such thing as a canola plant. Canola stands for "Canada Oil, Low Acid." It comes from rapeseed. To get rapeseed, corn or any other vegetable to the state of oil takes so much processing. That processing denatures, damages, and destroys the goodness of that initially naturally-occurring vegetable, seed, or grain. Denaturing and oxidizing fats make them very rancid and toxic for your cells.

These bad fats are very high in omega 6 fatty acids. Omega 6 acids are essential for the body, but the body can't use them if they are damaged and processed by man. Healthy omega 6 fats help build and protect your cells. Sources of omega 6's from bad fats clog up the cell, essentially blocking its front door. This cell congestion blocks the nutrients from getting in and toxins from getting out. The main nutrient that needs to get in to break down the barricaded doors is healthy omega 3 fatty acids. Omegas 3's balance out the bad omega 6's and unlock the cell. You get healthy omegas 3's and healthy omega 6's through healthy fats.

What are the good healthy fats? These are fats not altered by man and are any oil that occurs in nature in a real food state. Avocados, avocado oil, coconut, coconut oil, extra-virgin olive oil, olives, raw nuts, raw seeds, raw seed oils, real butter, and raw cheese. Grass-fed meats, free-range chicken, eggs, dairy, and wild-caught fatty fish are all great sources of healthy real fat.

MYTHS ABOUT FAT: GENETICS

Aren't these types of fats dangerous? Don't saturated fats cause heart disease? The truth is that heart disease is a sugar and bad-fat problem. I have a grandfather that passed away from heart disease. My father suffered from it. I have studied it greatly. Heart disease prevalence has exploded over the last 40 years. During that time, the low-fat and no-fat food craze exploded. We stripped the fat out of food, and all it did was make us fat and increase heart disease. There is no greater predictor of heart disease, high blood pressure, high cholesterol, and high triglycerides than the size of your waist! Your waist size is determined by your lifestyle as a sugar burner or a fat burner.

My parents and grandparents had heart disease and chronic disease--is fat what caused it? Everyone has good and bad genes. Bad genes are like a loaded gun. The genetics gun only goes off if you pull the trigger. Lifestyle is that trigger. Epigenetics is the study of what influences your good and your bad genes. You can reverse the risk of heart disease and other chronic diseases commonly blamed on genetics if you make the proper lifestyle improvements. The purpose of this book is to provide you with the actual solutions to do that.

You don't have to fear the genetics put inside of you. God did not mess up, and He did not give us real food designed to kill us. If man alters that good food and we don't take care of our bodies, then we pull the trigger.

> If you can "lifestyle" your way into it,
> you can "lifestyle" your way out of it.

The key to avoiding heart disease is controlling inflammation. Bad fat and sugar are gasoline for the fire. The amount of sugar and bad fats inside the blood damage the blood vessel. The body has to send a response, a scab, to repair the damage like a cut on your skin. That scab is cholesterol. Cholesterol forms inside of the arteries and repairs the cut. If you keep pounding sugar and bad fats in and damaging the blood vessels, more and more scar tissue builds up until the artery is clogged, which is a problem called coronary artery disease.

Sugar is the largest threat to your heart and overall health, but rancid, man-made, damaged fats also cause the same issue. Vegetable oil, cottonseed oil, canola oil, and others are all damaged fats that get into the system, and your body can't process them. These fats clog up your cells, leaving inflammation backed up in the system and toxins trapped in the cell. Those trapped toxins are the third primary cause of inflammation. The body has to respond with inflammation to try to flush them out but, because of the bad fats, the cell doors are blocked. In the next chapter we will break down how to clean up the toxins, but, first, let's dispel another myth about fat.

MYTHS ABOUT FAT: RED MEAT AND FAT CAUSE CHRONIC DISEASE

Another myth is that fat and red meat cause heart disease, cancer, osteoporosis, kidney disease, and other chronic diseases. Meat has been vilified recently, and I just don't believe that God put animals here on this planet to kill us. Now, everything should be in moderation, and if you do eat too much, it can be detrimental to your health; but healthy amounts of meat in your system can be a very good source of nutrients and healthy fats. If you are a vegetarian, more power to you--I don't think there's anything wrong with that. For some conditions, it's actually essential. I just want to make sure if you are a vegetarian that you're not eliminating meat and replacing it with sugar and toxic fake meat. I encounter lots of vegetarians that cut meat but replace it by eating pasta, bread, grains, rice, and soy products. I would rather you have a little bit of clean-sourced meat than take in all the excess sugars and bad fats.

The truth is that meat-eating societies have lived free of heart disease and cancers for centuries. You can study back thousands of years and find groups of people like Eskimos, for example, that lived strictly off fat and meat. No vegetables, no fruits, no grains, no carbohydrates--just pure fat and meat--yet they've thrived for thousands of years without higher incidences of chronic disease. Saturated fat from animal products is important at the cellular level, which is why it is in breast milk.

TOXIC BIOACCUMULATION: YOU ARE NOT WHAT YOU EAT--YOU ARE WHAT YOU EAT ATE

Not all meat is created equal. Meat can be very healthy but there are two major problems to watch out for. If you get too much of the bad stuff, you can really throw off your entire system. The first problem is toxic bioaccumulation. You are not what you eat--you are what you eat ate. Whatever is done to the animal is done to you. You are at the top of the food chain.

An insect eats bacteria or a small microorganism that has been exposed to chemicals. Then a small fish or a frog eats the insect that also came into contact with repellent. A larger fish eats the frog or eats the smaller fish, which also swam in water contaminated with fertilizer. Then a bird or a mammal eats the large fish that also received mercury exposure. You then end up eating the meat of the mammal or bird that also received vaccines and hormones.

This is toxic bioaccumulation. The bioaccumulation from the little bacteria all the way up to the animal that you finally eat carries a tremendous amount of toxicity. In fact, an herbivore like a cow that just feeds off plants or grains must eat 10 grams of living plants to make one gram of meat. It takes about five to eight pounds of chemically sprayed grain to produce one pound of beef.

(Growing up in Iowa) farmers would occasionally feed their cows candy in order to fatten them faster because they knew how much food it took just to produce one pound of beef. So if your cows are being fed toxic Skittles and chemically sprayed grain, they're not eating what they're designed to eat.

On top of that, the animals are pumped full of growth hormones to make them grow faster. This leads to a very sick animal. As the animal gets sick, it has to be given antibiotics and vaccinations. All the bad food, drugs, and sick animal meat end up in you. In fact, the primary sources of antibiotics that get into your system don't come from the doctor because you have an infection. They come from the meat that you're eating.

All of the same problems occur with chicken, too. If you are thinking I'll just stay away from meat and become a vegetarian or just eat seafood, hold on a second...

Not SOY fast! Soy has been often looked at as a great alternative to eating meat. You think you are getting a healthier meat substitute, but soy itself holds many hidden dangers. Soy is the most genetically-modified crop in America. Over 90% of it is genetically modified, and when you genetically modify food and eat it, you genetically modify yourself...

Soy can harm by mimicking estrogen inside of the body, which is a very bad thing because it increases prostate cancer in men and menopausal issues or breast cancer in women. Soy contains inhibitors that deter enzymes that are needed for breaking down protein inside your system, they can cause red blood cells to clump, they contain goitrogens which depress thyroid function, and they contain phytates which prevent absorption of minerals. If you are consuming soy, be sure it is non-GMO, but my advice is to use it sparingly.

Seafood has plenty of issues as well. Fish are now raised on farms (similar to cows and chickens), fed synthetic pellets, and given chemicals to help grow quickly. All of those chemicals can accumulate in you.

Pork and shellfish sit in the same class, as they are both bottom feeders. They eat whatever is in sight, leftovers and toxins alike. They're also very acidic, which tends to produce a lot more inflammation. If you eat the bottom feeder too often, then what does that make you?

The point is not to avoid eating meat; the point is to buy higher quality foods, changing the animal products you're eating first. Buying natural and organic meat is the biggest food- quality change you can make for the best return on the extra money it costs to buy it. Beef should be grass-fed, chicken free-range, fish wild-caught, and all three antibiotic- and hormone-free. You will radically reduce the toxic bioaccumulation effect. There is way more toxicity in a 2,000-pound cow than a head of broccoli. Spend the money on higher-quality meat first.

This goes for your supplements, too. For protein powder, I prefer collagen protein as it does not spike your insulin levels and put you into sugar-burning mode. This needs to be sourced from grass-fed cows. Fish oil supplements, which are great for reducing inflammation, must be sourced from wild-caught fish.

FATTY ACIDS: YOUR KEY TO REDUCING INFLAMMATION

Speaking of fish oil, let's discuss the second key that cleaning up your meat is going to do for you, which is balancing out the fatty-acid ratio in your body. Inside of you, there is a ratio of good, healthy fatty acids, primarily omega 6 and omega 3. As previously discussed, we get far too many toxic omega 6's through rancid fats, soybean oil, cottonseed oil, vegetable oil, and canola oil, as all of these bad oils are found inside of bread, grains, crackers, chips, etc. We get a huge dose of omega 6's, we don't get very many healthy omega 3's, and the gap between the 6's and the 3's is directly related to the inflammatory response inside of our body.

Your ideal ratio of omega 6 to omega 3 to reduce inflammation in the body is around 2:1. Interestingly enough, a grain-fed piece of beef has about a 20 to 1 ratio. A grass-fed piece of beef is the perfect 2:1 ratio. A healthy, well-fed animal means a healthy, well-fed you. Healthy amounts of omega 3, omega 6, and other fatty acids are a crucial weapon against the inflammation that is driving most chronic disease. Clean protein and proper fats like nuts, seeds, oils, and meats will supply you with the real food to fight back.

DON'T MAKE A GOOD FAT A BAD FAT

Man has a bad habit of making good healthy fats made by God into something bad. Overheating a good fat will damage all the good properties of the fat. If you have ever heated up oil such as olive oil or coconut oil and you've seen the oil smoke, you've now turned a good fat into bad fat. You make the fat rancid because at a certain point it can't tolerate being heated anymore. It's called the smoke point, and it represents the stability that the oil has, especially inside of your body.

Processed, man-made oils like vegetable oils have all been pushed past this smoke point in their production and made rancid before they even hit the shelf. Olive oil naturally occurs but has a low smoke point and should not be overheated. Coconut is the oil that we cook with in our house--it has a high smoke point and is very stable. Avocado does the same. Olive oil, which we use for salads and dressings, is the only other oil we have in the house. I would recommend only cooking with coconut or avocado oils as they have a very high smoke point and you have a very low chance of overheating them and making a good fat bad.

COOKWARE SO TOXIC IT WOULD KILL A BIRD

The other way to make a good fat bad is by cooking it in the wrong pan. If you, like millions of Americans, have non-stick cookware, then you may be causing your food and good fats a problem. Teflon and PFOAs are the problems with these pots and pans. Teflon pans, primarily made by DuPont, have been banned in European nations because they're directly linked to risks of liver, pancreatic, testicular and mammary gland tumors. They alter the thyroid hormone regulation, damage your immune system, and can affect fertility, birth, and the reproductive system. European nations have caught on to this and banned the toxin.

In America, millions of non-stick pans are still in use thanks to the profits of companies like DuPont. The main chemical in Teflon, PFOA, releases toxins at high temperatures and also flakes off into foods. If you've ever had a Teflon pan that starts flaking off over time, beware, because ingesting those flakes can be very harmful. One study just looked at the fumes from a Teflon pan that was exhausted into a birdcage, and it killed the bird. So if the fumes from PFOAs from a Teflon pan can kill a bird, imagine what it does to you, your children, or an unborn child?

Meat can be very good for the body, but there is no need to over-consume. Too much meat can cause issues, one being putting you into sugar-burning mode. There are two stop-checks if you're not losing weight or hitting your health goals. First, you may be consuming too much protein and your body is converting it into sugar. Decreasing protein sources, not fat, will throw you back into fat-burning mode. You don't need to cut it out completely, just don't overdo it.

The second roadblock to consider if you are struggling to lose weight or struggling to hit your health goals is addressing toxicity. That's exactly what we're going to cover in the next chapter because toxins are coming from all angles. You'll get a simple list that you can start to follow to radically reduce toxins by cleaning up the foods that you're eating.

5

CLEAN UP THE TOXINS

The third "C" of nutrition is to clean up the toxins. Our primary source of toxicity is the food that we're eating. In fact, the FDA has approved approximately 3,000 food additives, preservatives, and colorings that we're ingesting every day. The average person ingests 140 to 150 pounds of additives per year. We will break down the top 10 sources of toxins that you and your family can focus on eliminating from your diet to have the biggest impact on your toxin load.

1. CONDIMENTS AND DRESSINGS

Condiments and commercial salad dressings are loaded with bad fats, sugar, and a lot of toxins. They're made primarily with high fructose corn syrup and sugar so that you'll eat more of them. The bad fats come in the form of soybean oil, vegetable oil, cottonseed oil and other unrecognizable rancid fats.

These put you in sugar-burning mode and congest the cells with bad fats, and both in turn lead to inflammation. To make matters worse, most condiments and dressings have toxic additives like MSG (monosodium glutamate) which is a highly-addictive neurotoxin, which you'll soon learn about. Food colorings are added in to make the toppings look more appealing, and you'll soon learn just how bad these are for your health. If the condiment is fat-free, matters get worse because, if you take away the fat in any food, especially in condiments, you are adding in more sugar, and your body is less able to absorb the nutrients and the antioxidants from the salad, veggies, or food you put the topping on to begin with.

Check the door of your fridge. If you see things like soybean oil, canola oil, autolyzed yeast extract (MSG), food colorings, toxic preservatives, or just straight-up sugar added to your dressings and condiments, then they have to go. Check all your condiments while you are there and start replacing the most-used ones with healthy versions.

1. Make your own dressings from olive oil and vinegar or from the recipes in this book.
2. Find organic alternatives that do not contain rancid oils and toxins like MSG.
3. Load your salad up with extra nutrients if you do not have a healthy dressing by having your salad made of spinach, adding avocado, and putting olive oil on top.

2. CANDY

Well duh, Dr. Livingood. I know it seems kind of silly that the second toxin would be candy cause it's very obvious, but these little sugar bombs are loaded with high fructose corn syrup. High fructose corn syrup, if injected, will kill you quickly, but somehow if eaten through candy, doesn't. Maybe if it did we would stop eating so much! Fructose is terrible for your liver. When fructose hits the liver it instantly turns to triglycerides. That's right, candy directly increases your cholesterol levels and heart disease risk.

Nearly all candy contains bad oils and rancid fats, which congest the cells. They have absolutely no nutrition to them, so not only are they empty calories, but they block absorption of needed nutrients; yet we keep eating them because candy's sugar content is highly addictive, more so than narcotics, as we learned previously.

A Snickers bar is equivalent to seven teaspoons of sugar. One Hershey's dark chocolate bar is five and a half teaspoons of sugar. Every time you allow your kids to have one of these, you might as well just spoon several teaspoons of sugar directly into their mouth. No one would actually eat sugar by the spoonful, but until the craziness of putting candy in disgusts you, you'll never break the habit.

Candy is also loaded with dye so that it will look more appealing. Compounds in food dyes are linked to allergies, learning problems, hyperactivity, and mood disorders. Red dyes are considered a carcinogen but are still used in mass food production. They increase bladder cancer and tumors and are linked to thyroid cancer. Red 40, the most common dye, is found in candy, cereals, desserts, drugs and cosmetic products, and it is directly linked to allergies and ADHD in children.

Yellow #5 is currently undergoing testing, but has been linked to behavioral problems in kids and is found in many beverages, candy, cereals, gelatin, and pharmaceuticals. Yellow #6 is also undergoing testing, but it's been linked to adrenal tumors. Blue #1 is suspected of causing kidney tumors and is found in beverages, candy, cereals, and pharmaceuticals. Blue #2 increases the risk of tumors in the brain.

These food dyes may make our food look more appealing, but don't fall for the trick. Real food can be ugly as long as it puts nutrients into the system so you can experience real health.

1. Eliminate all candy during the Challenge Plan.
2. If you are to eat it, choose candies without red dyes and lots of bad oils.
3. Try the Livingood Daily Bars for a healthy candy bar.
4. Follow the recipes in the dessert section of this book to satisfy your sweet tooth.
5. Try stevia-sweetened chocolate to eliminate the sugar and still get your chocolate fix.

3. PACKAGED MEAT

To make our packaged meat look fresher, last longer, and be more addictive, they are loaded with chemicals. Nitrites are among the most dangerous additives. Nitrites are pumped into the meat to make it look bright red and fresh as well as to preserve the meat so it doesn't spoil and has a longer shelf life. The most common meat products containing nitrites are hot dogs, bacon, deli meats, sausage, pepperoni, beef jerky, frozen foods, and soups.

Nitrites are banned in many countries and were almost banned in the United States because the World Cancer Research Fund concluded in 2009 that many processed types of meat are too dangerous for human consumption. The University of Hawaii did a study that showed there's a 67% risk of pancreatic cancer with high nitrite exposure. They've also been linked to altering DNA and causing developmental issues in children of pregnant mothers eating a lot of red meat that contains nitrites.

1. Choose nitrite-free and natural or organic processed meats.
2. Try safer alternatives to bacon and hotdogs like turkey bacon or chicken sausage.

4. BREADS AND GRAINS

Next on the toxin list are bread and grains, especially white bread. Bread and grain in its real, whole, natural form is not bad for us in moderation and can actually be nutritious. Man has messed up another real food. Bread commonly starts off with chemically-sprayed grain. To make white bread, the minerals, nutrients, and fiber is stripped from the grain and bleached. On top of bad sugars, the bleached grain is combined with bad fats like soybean oil and preservatives to make white bread. These anti-nutrients have to be fortified with synthetic vitamins to salvage the food. When white bread hits the body, it immediately turns into sugar in the mouth and causes a tremendous spike in blood sugar and insulin levels. Watch out for the diabetes sandwich.

Grains in their whole, real form that are used to make bread, pasta, tortillas, chips, crackers, and other products can be eaten healthy, if done at the right time in the right moderation. Here are the guidelines for bread and grains.

1. Avoid white bread and grain products.
2. Avoid wheat-based products, especially those high in gluten and sugars.
3. Look for whole grain, sprouted, or seed-based bread, crackers, chips, tortillas, pasta, and other grain-based products.
4. Beware of rancid oils that leave the body congested added to grain-based products.
5. Avoid oats, grains, cereals, bread, crackers, chips, tortillas, and other high-carbohydrate, grain-based products until completing the Challenge Plan and hitting your health goals.
6. Avoid oats, grains, cereals, bread, crackers, chips, tortillas, and other carbohydrates ending in -ose. Grain-based products can be enjoyed in moderation on the Everyday Plan if sourced from organic, whole-grain sources.
7. Try almond, coconut, and/or cassava root-based bread, flours, chips, crackers, tortillas, and desserts in this book as alternatives in order to stay in fat-burning mode.

5. SPRAYED PRODUCE

Next is sprayed produce. Every year, three million pesticides are used around the world. There are no disclosures on the produce of what pesticides you're taking in, so you don't even know what you're eating. Many of the chemicals that are being used on the produce to kill bugs and prolong the life of produce have never been studied for long-term effects on human beings. The regulations are very loose, and you get an average of 70 exposures to toxic pesticides daily.

Overall, pesticides greatly increase the toxic load on your body. Pesticide exposure itself has been directly linked to nervous system disorders, immune system suppression, allergic reactions, childhood cancers, breast cancers, diabetes, reproductive damage, hormonal problems, asthma, exacerbation of ADD and ADHD, autism, migraine headaches, and growth and developmental delays. In fact,

Round Up producer Monsanto is in multiple lawsuits because their product contains high levels of glyphosate. Glyphosate destroys the gut, which makes up 80% of the immune system. This has been directly linked to cancer, as proven recently in a class-action $100 million lawsuit proving a man's lymphoma was caused by the toxic pesticide. This has opened the door for many other victims to step forward.

If one of the largest companies in the world is forced to pay millions of dollars because it is proven in a court of law that the pesticide they use on your fruits and vegetables causes cancer, then that is grounds to switch your food to organic. Typically, organic produce is going to reduce the toxic load on the system because pesticides, especially the very harmful ones, are not used on organic produce.

In 2006, a study published in the Journal of Environmental Health Perspectives reported that children fed a diet of organic vegetables have six to nine times fewer pesticides in their urine and in their bloodstream than those that were eating processed foods. Organic produce not only reduces the toxin load, but it has a higher nutrient level. In fact, a study out of the Journal of American Agricultural and Food Chemistry found that organically-grown fruits and vegetables contain higher levels of cancer-fighting antioxidants than conventional pesticide-sprayed produce. You might not be able to buy all of your foods organic, but it would be worth spending extra to buy organic to replace the ones which contain the most toxins.

The Clean 15/Dirty Dozen

The Environmental Working Group created this list to show the "dirty" 12 foods that you always want to get organic because their skin is thin and they tend to absorb higher levels of pesticides. The "clean" list of 15 fruits and vegetables are the produce you can get conventional and you don't have to worry about buying organic because they have tough skin, which naturally repels the pesticides that were used to grow them. If buying all foods organic is too expensive, then save on groceries by buying at least the Dirty Dozen foods organic.

Clean 15	Dirty Dozen
Sweet corn	Strawberries
Avocados	Spinach
Pineapples	Nectarines
Cabbage	Apples
Onions	Peaches
Frozen Sweet Peas	Pears
Papayas	Cherries
Asparagus	Grapes
Mangos	Celery
Eggplant	Tomatoes
Honeydew	Sweet Bell Peppers
Kiwi	Potatoes
Cantaloupe	
Cauliflower	
Grapefruit	

6. MARGARINE AND SYNTHETIC BUTTER

The sixth toxin is the man-made butter alternative, margarine. Long touted as a great replacement for its real-food counterpart butter, margarine continues to populate America's refrigerators' despite its toxic makeup. Margarine has a similar chemical structure to plastic and is made up of dangerous rancid oils that congest the cells and cause inflammation.

Here's a clip from Nourishing Traditions by Sally Fallon on how margarine is made:Here's a clip from Nourishing Traditions by Sally Fallon on how margarine is made:

"Manufacturers begin with the cheapest oils, soy, corn, cottonseed or canola, already rancid from the extraction process, and mix them with tiny metal particles, usually nickel oxide. The oil with its nickel catalyst is then subjected to hydrogen gas in a high-pressure, high-temperature reactor. Next, soap-like emulsifiers and starch are squeezed into the mixture to give it a better consistency. The oil is yet again subjected to high temperatures when it is deemed clean. This removes the unpleasant odor. Margarine's natural color is an unappetizing gray, and it's removed by bleach. Dyes and strong flavors must then be added to make it resemble butter. And finally, the mixture is compressed andpackaged in blocks or tubs and sold as health-food."

As you can see by this detailed production description, margarine is far from health food and incredibly toxic. So what should you use? Butter. Real butter is good for the system. It is unprocessed and contain healthy fats and nutrients that actually help your brain and body decrease inflammation. In fact, if you were to do an experiment today and put margarine, reduced fat butter, and normal butter on a plate and set it outside, ants would actually be smarter than many Americans. Ants would actually go and eat the natural butter first and avoid the synthetic and plastic forms like margarine. Use the real stuff. It's closer to nature, and it's good for your body as a whole.

1. Discontinue the use of margarine and all synthetic or low-fat butter and oils.
2. Use real organic, grass-fed, or raw butter.
3. Olive, coconut, avocado, and grapeseed oil products can be used as long as they do not contain additional rancid oils.

7. TOXIC DRINKS

Number 7 is toxic drinks. We, of course, know that sugary, man-made drinks are very detrimental to our health. Diet sodas and sugar-free products might be even worse. Diet and sugar-free products contain high amounts of aspartame and Splenda. We discussed these extensively in the sugar chapter, but these excitotoxins excite the cells of your brain to the point of cell death. Most people eat them to try to lose weight, but, as research shows, people who use diet products actually gain more weight because these diet products increase appetite. With sugar products out and toxic artificial sweeteners out, what can you focus on drinking?

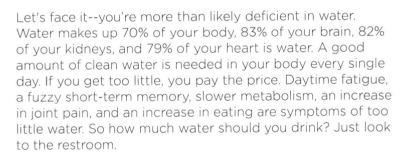

1. Avoid all sugary sodas, teas, and drinks.
2. Try stevia-sweetened soda like Zevia as a better alternative.
3. Avoid diet or sugar-free anything.
4. Avoid "health drinks" like Gatorade and Vitamin Water that are loaded with sugar, dyes, and toxins.
5. Organic coffee and tea.
6. Sparkling water without artificial flavors or sugar.
7. Use greens powder in your water for better absorption.
8. Drink water and try adding fresh lemon, lime, cucumbers, or other nutrient infusers.

Everything You Need to Know About Water

Let's face it--you're more than likely deficient in water. Water makes up 70% of your body, 83% of your brain, 82% of your kidneys, and 79% of your heart is water. A good amount of clean water is needed in your body every single day. If you get too little, you pay the price. Daytime fatigue, a fuzzy short-term memory, slower metabolism, an increase in joint pain, and an increase in eating are symptoms of too little water. So how much water should you drink? Just look to the restroom.

The more yellow your urine is, the more water you need. If you have clear urine, then you're in the clear and you're drinking enough. Drink water slowly throughout the day. A water sprinkler slowly saturates the grass of a yard so the soil can slowly be saturated. A bucket of water on the yard just runs right off, and much less soaks into the soil. Your water intake should mimic the sprinkler, slow saturation every 10-15 minutes throughout the day. Consume half of your body weight in ounces in fresh water daily; however, not all water is created equal.

When it comes to the right type of water to drink, it's a loaded question. To get proper water into the system, be sure it is filtered to minimize toxins. Drink half of your body weight in ounces of water per day, but use Greens and minerals to drive that water into your cells because it's not how much you drink, it's how much you absorb. There is also the issue of acidity. Let's take a look at the purity, acidity, and energy of water.

1. WATER PURITY AND FILTRATION

According to the Environmental Working Group, over 260 contaminants have been found in our nation's tap water supply and more than half of them have no safety standards at all. There are 78 chemicals used in industrial and consumer products and 52 additives that are linked to cancer. Chemicals in local tap water include gasoline, percolates from rocket fuel, arsenic, lead, chlorine, fluoride, hormone-disrupting phthalates, and coal.

Potentially the biggest issue with unfiltered water is pharmaceuticals. Every time you flush drugs down the toilet or throw one in the garbage, you are potentially impacting and toxifying everyone else around you. Most tap water contains cholesterol drugs, pain relievers, and mental health medications.

Water filtration is a must. For obvious reasons, tap water would be the worst to drink. A good start would be to get bottled water, a fridge filter, or pitcher filter. Bottled water at least has filtration but the downfall is large companies like Coke and Pepsi now produce a lot of them with poor health standards. Minimal house filtration will at least pull out toxins like chloride and microbes, but still does not touch the drugs and other chemicals.

Reverse osmosis would be the next level up in water filtration. It takes out almost all of the chemicals, including the drugs. This leaves the water pure, but the downfall is that it may leave the water demineralized and "deadened." The filtration strips out the minerals that get the water into the cells and can also make the water more acidic. We will touch on this in a moment.

The optimal way I have found to remove all the impurities and chemicals, including fluoride, is to use high surface area filtration. The downfall is it is more expensive. This more gentle approach to filtration puts the water in contact with chemical absorbing organic compounds to pull out the impurities without pulling out all the minerals and energy and making it acidic. Having this attached to your sink would be a step up, and my family and I use this form as a whole house filtration unit, which is ideal.

2. ACIDITY AND WATER

Are you drinking acid water? The pH in your body must maintain a balance to keep you in a disease-fighting, anti-inflammatory state. When your body becomes too acidic from the food we eat like sugar, alcohol, processed foods, and bad fats, then it is in a disease-forming state. Many forms of water, especially bottled waters, are very acidic. Diseases like cancer love acid.

Spring water traditionally has a healthier alkaline level. This just makes sense--it's in the form God made it. Just like real food, it's real water. Now, man can make good water bad by exposing it to chemicals. Always shoot for your water being in a glass container to eliminate the chemicals like the reproductive- system disrupting phthalates that leach into the water from plastics. Investigate the source and company that produces your favorite spring water to get the best quality.

Some remedy the acid problem with highly alkaline water. It is not quite that simple. I would advise water to be alkaline, but not too much. Too much alkalinity, just like too much acidity, can also cause damage. Bleach, for example, is alkaline and can cause damage. Too much highly alkaline water poured into your digestive tract can weaken it over time. Your stomach has a pH of 2-3. Pouring pH 9.5 water in it all the time can weaken its strength and protective mechanisms. The same goes for distilled water.

Alkaline and distilled water are very useful tools in the natural remedy of disease, I just don't believe it is natural to be drinking them all the time. Healing skin ailments, overcoming sickness, and detoxing are the best uses for distilled and alkaline water. On a daily basis, shoot for water that is slightly alkaline like spring or surface area filtered.

Eat real food rather than processed, which is the cause of the acidity in the first place, and drink your water as real as possible.

3. ENERGY AND MINERALS AND WATER

Water has life to it. A flowing stream babbling from the ground has energy and nutrition to it. That energy gives you life. A stagnant pond that does not move has no energy and much more toxicity to it. Which would you rather drink? Water that is under-filtered or over-filtered loses its energy and its nutrients. To have the healthiest water, step three is to re-mineralize and re-energize the water.

As with any of these steps, there are multiple levels for improving the nutrition and energy of your water. The one that has been the most effective for me is adding greens to my water. It is not about how much water you drink, but how much you absorb.

A while back, I had a microscopic blood work test (which is blocked for use in the United States) to test the health of my cells. Healthy cells=healthy you. I was drinking the recommended amount of half your body weight in ounces daily, but I found out that the water was running off instead of soaking in. My water needed minerals to help direct it. Minerals like potassium help direct water into cells.

I learned greens powder was the easiest, most convenient way to do it, so I created my own. I loaded it with spirulina, chlorella, enzymes, fruits, and other superfoods to drive in the water, drive down the inflammation, and give my body an easy way to get nutrients. Nothing replaces real food, but this is as close as I can get on days when I barely get a lunch break. This one change fixed the absorption problem 100% on my follow-up testing.

I occasionally add sea salt to my water and diet to help support that lack of minerals in my body as well. If food and bad water are depleting these minerals, then real sea salt and greens are the best and safest way to counteract it.

The final advice concerning water is to consume it when it is most alive. How does water get energy? Think stagnant pond water and flowing stream. Water gets energy through movement. For this reason, simply swirling your water before drinking it adds life. If you are dealing with a chronic disease you can get a water energizer. It uses a vortex to spin life back into your water. Our family goes to the extreme and uses this to re-energize the water, but it does not (step) one in the journey to real health. Let me lay out the priority order for healthy water.

1. Consume half of your body weight in ounces of fresh water daily.
2. Consume filtered or bottled water. Spring and slightly alkaline are best.
3. Add greens powder and/or minerals to your water for higher absorption and energy.
4. Drink from glass instead of plastic to avoid toxicity.
5. Get a kitchen filtration system.
6. Get a whole house filtration system.
7. Get a water re-mineralizer or re-energizer.

Salt and Potassium

According to a 1985 article in the New England Journal of Medicine entitled "Paleolithic Nutrition," our ancient ancestors got about 11,000 mg of potassium a day and only about 700 mg of sodium. Today, this equates to nearly 16 times more potassium than sodium. Compare that to our SAD (Standard American Diet); today we on average consume only about 2,500 mg of potassium daily. The conservative recommended daily allowance is 4,700 mg, so we're even well-below that. The second problem is that we are not only getting significantly lower amounts of potassium compared to our ancestors, but also that we are consuming on average 3,600 mg of sodium.

This may also explain why high-sodium diets appear to affect some people but not others. We don't have a sodium problem in this country. We have a potassium problem. In fact, a 2006 study in the American Journal of Medicine compared the daily sodium intake of 78 million Americans to the risk of dying from heart disease over the course of 14 years. The study concluded that lower-sodium diets lead to higher mortality rates among those with cardiovascular disease, which raises questions regarding the likelihood of a survival advantage on a low-sodium diet.

Now certainly you should not hear that you can eat lots of salt, it's the type of salt you eat that is key. Your body needs real salt, the kind God made that is full of minerals and nutrients, not the toxic table salt found in packaged foods in high amounts. Shop to the outside of the store, limit your processed foods intake and put proper potassium and sodium in through real food, fruits, and vegetables. When you follow the Make Food Simple plans with real salt and lots of real foods, your ratios of potassium and sodium start resembling your ancestors.

When I mention potassium, most people think of a banana, but green juices and vegetables contain even healthier amounts. In fact, spinach has two times as much potassium than bananas. If you focus on vegetables, you'll get enough in. As for salt, you want the real stuff, not table salt--that's toxic. Celtic or Himalayan Sea salt is God's version of electrolytes. Not man-made toxic, sugary Gatorade. The salt you use should contain 50+ minerals and electrolytes. Don't be scared of real salt: your body needs it. Be scared of processed, man-made food and all the preservatives that come with it.

A cheat that I use on a daily basis to get extra potassium, vegetables, and minerals into my system is through greens powder. Daily greens powder is an easy way to add additional vegetables to an already great nutrition plan. With extra nutrients and servings of things like spinach, kale, chlorella, spirulina, broccoli, turmeric, enzymes, and probiotics, your body will drive nutrients and water into your cells for detox and energy. Healthy cells equal a healthy you.

1. Use high-quality Celtic or Himalayan sea salt regularly on food and in water to re-mineralize your body.
2. Avoid table salt (NaCl) and processed salts found in packaged foods.
3. Increase potassium intake through juicing, eating real fruits and vegetables, and greens powder.

8. GENETICALLY MODIFIED FOOD

Number eight on the toxicity list is genetically modified foods. This topic is very easy for me to discuss, so it won't take us long. This violates the major premise of the Make Food Simple plan. Eat real food. It does not matter much to me that the science is still needed to make big conclusions about how bad for us GMO food really is, because for me it is simple. If God made it, eat it. If He didn't, don't. Man's altering the genetic makeup of food just doesn't sound like a good idea.

The most prevalent genetically-modified foods that you can eat are soybeans and corn, as over 90% of the American supply of soybeans and corn are now genetically modified. These crops are genetically modified to allow for major pesticide use so that insects around the crop can be killed, but not the actual crop. Unlike packaged foods, these processed plants do not come with any warning labels.

The American Academy of Environmental Medicine States that several animal studies have indicated serious health risks associated with genetically modified foods causing immune problems, infertility, accelerated aging, faulty insulin regulation and changes in major organs like the gastrointestinal system. They're asking physicians to advise patients to avoid genetically modified foods.

If you alter the DNA of a food and then you eat the altered DNA, what do you think will happen to your DNA?

Choose local, natural, and/or organic produce when possible to increase nutrients and avoid genetically modified foods. Also, look at the 4 to 5-digit code on any produce and vegetables that you purchase to find out if it is genetically modified. A simple guide is below:

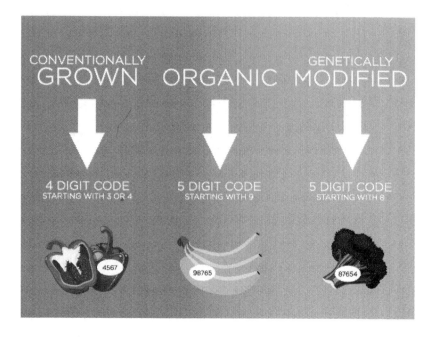

9. COMMERCIAL DAIRY

Number nine on the toxic food list is commercial dairy. The "Milk, It does a body good" marketing campaign was one of the most toxic food crazes to ever hit America. Milk and dairy in their real-food, raw form, may do a body good, but man-made milk does not. My grandpa was a dairy farmer in Iowa, and I grew up drinking milk with every meal. Milk was labeled as a health food, but--spoiler alert--I am about to ruin your thoughts on consuming commercial dairy.

In 1971 an average cow produced 9,700 pounds of milk per year. With the 1990s "Milk, It does a body good" campaigns, there was a milk-demand explosion. This forced farmers to up production and cut corners to maintain a profit. The corners they cut were your health.

The average cow now produces 19,000 pounds of milk in a year. To produce two times the amount of milk, the cow must be loaded with growth hormone. As the cow grows faster and is milked more, it gets sick. Just like you or I would if we doubled our workload and put on 40 pounds of steroid muscle.

When the cow is sick it has to be loaded with vaccinations and antibiotics to keep it alive to produce milk. Twenty-four hours a day, these cows are taken on and off the milk production machines. This produces sores. The sores give off pus. The FDA currently allows 750,000,000 pus cells per liter of milk in the United States. Yes, you read that correctly, 750 MILLION pus cells.

To counteract the pus, commercial dairy is flash-heated, or pasteurized. When heated to high temperatures, the nutrients and proteins that are the benefit in dairy products in the first place are destroyed. Commercial dairy is loaded with antibiotics, growth hormones, vaccinations, and a considerable amount of pus, but its nutrients are destroyed. How it ever became a health food is beyond me, but it is just not worth it.

Our family pretty much avoids milk. The only sources of dairy we consume now are raw cheese, grass-fed butter, organic sour cream, and occasionally organic cottage cheese or organic half-and-half for coffee. Dairy can be consumed, but it is grossly--pun intended--over-consumed.

1. Stay away from commercial dairy.
2. Use hormone-free, antibiotic free, and organic options. Raw, especially for cheese, whenever possible.
3. Use alternative, minimally-processed, plant-based products like almond milk, cashew milk, coconut milk or oat milk products.

10. PACKAGED FOOD

Number 10 on the toxic list is seasoned packaged foods. The foods on the inside aisles of the store, packaged foods, are full of toxins. This is why you must start doing your shopping on the outside aisles of the store where the majority of the real food is. Pasta, rice mixes, soup mixes, snack chips, crackers, bread, dressings, canned meals, and frozen meals are all loaded with preservatives, dyes, and chemicals for taste. Since we have already discussed dyes and toxic salt preservatives, let's focus on one of the most toxic food additives monosodium glutamate, MSG.

We've mentioned it a couple of times leading up to this point, but it was discovered in 1908 in China and introduced in the United States in 1948. It very quickly became a multibillion-dollar industry. Its toxin potential was first discovered in the 1960's.

The danger with MSG is it is an excitotoxin. This means it has carcinogenic properties that excite cells, especially neurons (brain cells), to the point of death. Most people are allergic to it and some have severe allergic reactions. Symptoms include headaches, migraines, fertility issues, mood swings, depression, hyperactivity, asthma, heart irregularities, and hormone disruption.

Now that the world is starting to catch on to the fact that MSG is toxic, food producers have started hiding it in our food. Here are code names for MSG:

Always Contain MSG	May Contain MSG
Monosodium glutamate	Maltodextrin
Potassium glutamate	Malt extract
Autolyzed yeast	Bouillon/broth/stock
Yeast extract	Natural or Artificial flavoring
Yeast food	Natural beef/chicken flavoring
Yeast nutrient	Seasoning or Spices
Hydrolyzed vegetable protein	Soy sauce
Hydrolyzed protein	Soy protein isolate/concentrate
Hydrolyzed plant protein	Whey protein isolate
Hydrolyzed oat flour	Gelatin
Plant protein extract	Carrageenan
Sodium caseinate	Enzyme modified
Calcium caseinate	Protein fortified
Textured protein	Ultra-pasteurized

The point is MSG needs to be avoided. If you love your brain and you like the neurons of your body, MSG and packaged food have to go. Many other good alternatives are around, so what do you do?

You avoid the toxins on the Toxic Top 10 list and start finding alternatives.

1. Condiments and Dressings. You can make your own. You can use things like olive oil, avocado oil, coconut oil to mix up your own dressings. There are several recipes in this book for sauces and dressings to do exactly that.
2. Candy. You just need to kick the habit; there are some great ice cream, cooky, and dessert recipes in this book so that you can make healthy versions of these without the bad fats and all the toxic sugars.
3. Packaged Meats: Start purchasing deli and packaged meats from natural or organic sources to cut down on the nitrite, antibiotic, and toxic preservative consumption.
4. White Bread. Choose whole, sprouted, or stone ground wheat or seeded bread. If you are on the Challenge Plan, you need to avoid this all together until your goals are hit.
5. Sprayed produce. Follow the Clean 15/Dirty Dozen lists and learn how to shop to eliminate the toxic loads for you and your family.
6. Margarine and Synthetic Butter. Use butter straight-up. It and other real oils like olive oil are fantastic for you.
7. Toxic Drinks. Drink water, half of your body weight in ounces on a daily basis. Tea and green tea are other options as well as the Greens powder to help you absorb the water in the first place. If you absolutely have to have a soda, reach for Zevia, which is Stevia-sweetened soda.
8. Genetically Modified Foods. These need to be eliminated by focusing on all-natural and organic produce.
9. Commercial Dairy. Should be replaced with organic or raw dairy. Start using alternatives like coconut and almond milk.
10. Packaged Foods. Start shopping on the outside aisles of the store and focus on organic and natural alternatives.

The focus is on real food. The more you cook it and/or process it, the fewer nutrients and the more toxicity it contains. We have a lot of amazing food to eat on this earth. You are not going to starve. We have disease from excess food while other countries have disease from too little. Most of us could stand to skip a few meals anyway. By making food simple, you can change your taste buds and learn to love real food.

Nothing tastes as good as health feels.

6

CARE ABOUT NUTRIENTS AND CURB CONSUMPTION

Let's review the 5 C's of Making Food Simple:

1. Cut the sugar.
2. Crank up good fat.
3. Clean up the toxins.
4. Care about nutrients.
5. Curb your consumption.

We have covered the first three, which is the bulk of healthy eating. Let's break down the fourth and fifth C's where we will get you and your family to care about nutrients and reveal your secret weapon to health restoration by curbing your consumption.

CARE ABOUT NUTRIENTS

Grocery Shopping

We simply do not get enough nutrients into our system. This chapter is all about eating to live instead of living to eat. Caring about nutrients is a huge part, and it all starts with shopping. Let's turn you into a sharp, smart grocery shopper.

Number one, you have to plan. Have you ever gone to the grocery store hungry with no list? You leave with six treats or snacks you normally wouldn't buy and two meals that will go to waste because, although they sounded good, you won't actually cook them. Focused time in the store is set up with a proper list and planned time to get in and get out before those cookies and chips suck you in!

Schedule your shopping time for the week. Our family shops at the grocery store at the same time every Sunday after church. We make, or should I say my wife makes, a list of exactly what we need. We divide the list and each takes a kid or two. (Have you ever tried to grocery shop with three toddlers? It will make you eat sugar!) Most of our shopping is done in the produce, nuts, meats, and egg/cheese sections. We grab a few items from the middle of the store, our 4-year-old and 2-year-old eat a half a bag of grapes while we do this--that saves a couple of dollars and we are out!

The key is that we pick 2-4 meals from this book before we go in. We simply write down (or have memorized) the ingredients of our favorite meals and make a list. Our pantry is typically stocked with the needed spices, condiments, and add-ins to make these meals go. Coconut milk, cinnamon, amino acids, and almond flour are examples of a few food pantry staples (Check out the Pantry List in the book to see them all).

We don't have to get those pantry staples each week. So trip one is a little heavier, but once we get in a groove of the 10-15 meals we like during each season of the year, we pretty much rotate those through our meal plan each week and have the needed staples on hand.

We keep it simple. I swear our kids live off berries, hummus, veggies, organic deli meat, chicken, black beans, eggs, and smoothies. No milk. They drink water, greens, and sparkling water. No candy. We make desserts from this book or have one of my bars. Their meals are quick and oftentimes don't need heating. Occasionally we try a new recipe, but if it isn't quick and fun to make, or is not really well-received, we don't add it to our favorites.

1. Pick your favorite recipes from the book and make a list. Plan!
2. Shop to the outside of the store
3. Spend extra on animal products first, then the dirty dozen list, and finally all other foods natural or organic.
4. Ideally, get fresh produce. The second best is frozen. Third, and least desired, is canned food.
5. Read every ingredient label.

Shopping On a Budget

Come prepared--I can't stress this enough. We always have a list to know what we're going to be buying. That saves us money because we usually stick just to the list so quality food can be the priority, not filler foods. Eating healthy can actually save you money in the long run because if you can plan ahead and use the recipes from the book, you can be planning out meals and getting quality food, meaning that you don't have to be going out to eat or spending money on junk food.

You can't buy back your health. Once it's gone, it's gone. If there were one thing to spend more on, it would be your food, supplements, and health. It's the best investment you can make. If you think you cannot afford it, then consider this: you cannot afford not to. You can't afford heart disease, cancer, or kidney failure. Health care cost is the number one cause of bankruptcy in America. Plus, if you just took all that money you are spending on soda, candy, junk food, fast food, alcohol, and eating out, you would be able to afford it.

Another tip for shopping smart and saving on produce is to buy fresh and in season. Buying local cuts down on shipping and delivery costs to save you money. To prevent wasting money, buy fruits and vegetables only two to three days at a time so they don't spoil. Find out what's in season in your area by googling your state's in-season produce online. Try to source your vegetables and your fruits as local as possible because they're going to have a higher nutrient content. To find these easier, consider shopping at places like farmer's markets, co-ops, and health food stores.

My family also throws in a trip to a bulk food store every few weeks. Shopping at stores like Costco or Sam's Club can really help you save. We buy bulk nuts, berries, meat, eggs, coconut oil, sparkling water, and green juice because we eat so much of them and it helps us save.

Consider splitting large meat orders with friends or family to save on higher quality meat. Look for deals and coupons online. Food delivery and online bulk orders are becoming more and more prominent.

Grow your own food in the garden. When I was a kid growing up in Iowa, we had a huge garden full of delicious vegetables. Even if you only have a back porch, you can still have some planted veggies. Not only does it save, but also it is hard to beat the taste.

Final quick budget tips are to reduce eating out by planning ahead and eating in with your family. Make food and meals fun. Try Friday homemade pizza night, make your own taco salad night, wing night, BBQ night, Asian food night, etc.

The primary focus, if you are on a tight budget, is to change your animal products first. Spend more on organic and natural meats because there's way more toxicity in a 2,000-pound cow, than there is in a head of broccoli. If you are buying produce organic, focus on the dirty dozen list first, and then on everything else being natural or organic if it is in your budget.

Label Reading Is A Must

Look for the minimal number of ingredients possible. An apple only has one ingredient--less is better. Look for real ingredients. If you can't pronounce it, it's probably not that good for you. Try to buy more foods without any labels at all, like fruits and vegetables. Check every single label on every product you buy.

Over time, you're going to learn what to get and what not

to get in the stores where you shop. For healthy shopping, avoid at all costs man-made ingredients on the labels. Focus on the ingredient list more than the nutrition label. The serving sizes and nutrition facts can be manipulated and skewed. This is one common form of questionable food marketing. The second is the use of health buzzwords like made with real ingredients, trans-fat-free, fat-free, enriched, natural flavors, or sugar-free. These all usually raise red flags and need investigating. The ingredients label will reveal the truth.

The third most common form of questionable marketing on foods is endorsements. For example, the American Heart Association has companies that pay them to put their logo on a food product. The questionable part comes in when the logo is on a product like a grain or cereal bar. Many of these products that are endorsed contain toxic sugar and bad oils that have been shown to cause heart disease.

Here's a short list of the major culprits to look for and avoid in every foods' main ingredients:

Any form of Monosodium Glutamate (Hydrolyzed, autolyzed, yeast extract, etc)

Any form of Sugar (Fructose, sucrose, corn syrup, maltodextrin, etc.)

Any Rancid Oil or Fat (Hydrogenated, cottonseed, vegetable, soybean, canola, etc)

Any Artificial Sweetener (Aspartame, Splenda, sucralose, NutraSweet, etc)

Any Refined, White Flours and Grains (Wheat, enriched flour, corn, malt, bran, etc)

Any Additives, Colorings, Preservatives, and Other Chemicals (Red 40, TBHQ, benzoates, salts, etc)

SUPPLEMENTATION IS NOT JUST A RECOMMENDATION, IT IS NOW A REQUIREMENT

Our food and soil are losing their nutrient supply. Unless you are eating all of your food straight out of your own nutrient-dense soil in your garden, then chances are you are not getting the nutrients you need. When comparing the content of 13 different nutrients found in 43 crops, scientists found that on average, the soil content has declined 6% to 38% for different nutrients in our soil over the last 100 years. You have to eat more fruits and veggies to get the nutrients you need. So supplementation is not just a recommendation, it is a requirement.

Supplements still need to follow the same rules as real food. Many people make this mistake. All day long, I analyze supplements for patients, and I consistently see the same mistakes. After 25,000+ patients, here are the most common supplement mistakes:

1. Cut the Sugar. Just like in food, rule number one is violated often. Especially powdered supplements, but pill form, too. Watch out for whey proteins, corn, maltodextrin, and any form of fructose or sugar names we have discussed.
2. Crank Up the Good Fat. Which means remove the bad fat. Poor quality supplements are loaded with soybean oils and rancid fish oils.
3. Clean up the Toxins. As discussed with food, supplements have some common toxins.
    - Magnesium Stearate
    - Toxic Dyes (Red 40, Blue 2, etc)
    - Titanium Dioxide
    - Soy
    - Whey Protein From Non-Grass-Fed Cows
    - Whey Isolate (Highly Processed and Contains Heavy Metals)
4. Care About Nutrients. Supplement ingredients made from real foods with no gluten, wheat, dairy, or genetically modified foods are crucial. Just like with the guidelines of food we want high-quality real ingredients in supplements.

5. Vitamin D. Vitamin D2 is synthetic vitamin D that is often prescribed. D3 is a healthy form. Every 1000 iu of vitamin D must be taken with 100 mg of vitamin K to prevent calcification of the arteries. Vitamin D is fat-soluble and should be taken with a healthy fat for better absorption.

6. Omegas. To protect quality should be in non-see-through containers with less than 120 capsules. Watch out for toxic additives, colorings, and bad fats. A high dose of Omega 3s to cut down inflammation and healthy Omega 6, 7, and 9s are a plus. Antioxidants should be added to protect the oil's quality.

7. Multi-Vitamins. Avoid toxic additives, colorings, and sugars. If containing B vitamins, be sure they are the methyl forms to avoid sensitivity issues to non-methylated forms like folic acid.

8. Greens. Make sure the greens contain no sugars or forms of sugar ending in -ose, maltodextrin, or the toxic additives above. Ideally should be dairy-, GMO-, and wheat-free. As organic as possible with a wide range of fruits, veggies, and nutrients.

9. Collagen. Collagen does not spike insulin levels like other protein powders. Collagen depletes with age, so it is needed to support the skin, hair, and nails, and to repair the gut and joints. Be sure it is sourced from grass-fed, free-range animals. Be sure there are no added sugars.

10. Probiotics. Make sure they do not contain fillers and toxins. They must be in a stable form so they don't spoil or are killed before they get deep into your gut. You can get most of these by eating raw vegetables and fermented food like sauerkraut, kombucha, kefir, and apple cider vinegar. I get mine through foods and the greens powder.

11. Calcium. Most people do not need calcium supplementation; they need mineral balance. Science suggests to not take more than 600mg per day, especially if you have heart and blood vessel issues. For bone strength, it should be taken with magnesium, vitamin D, and vitamin K.

12. Other supplements to consider are vitamin C, turmeric, and magnesium.

Don't just take supplements, ask us or someone with the knowledge to help consolidate and save on exactly what would benefit you personally. If you begin taking too many supplements for vague reasons, you can just end up with expensive bathroom breaks because the excess nutrients may be just going right through you. Remember, it's not how much you take--it is how much you absorb. High-quality, targeted nutrients made from real food are worth the extra dollars.

I believe one of the best supplements you can take on a daily basis is a greens powder. We significantly lack vegetables and fruits, and if the greens powder is high enough quality, it can replace several supplements in one. Vitamin D, Omegas, and Collagen Protein are the other three that most Americans could benefit from. Nutrients are best-absorbed and used through food. Nothing replaces a good diet, but instead of turning to drugs, high-quality supplements can be a great approach to dealing with conditions and experiencing real health.

CURB YOUR CONSUMPTION

The fifth "C" of nutrition is to curb your consumption. Let's face it: we eat way too much. Americans have been sold the lie that we need to eat three to six times a day, but when you think about our ancestors 1,000 years ago, they might have been lucky if they ate every couple of days. We now eat breakfast at 6:00 am, a snack at 10:00 am, a big lunch at noon, a soda or sugar drink at 3:00 pm, a big dinner at 6:00 pm, we munch in front of the TV before bed and occasionally sneak to the kitchen or through a drive-thru after midnight to feed our addiction.

No wonder we are overweight and chronically ill. One of the best things you can possibly do to heal your body is to curb your consumption. If your body is not expending energy processing food, it's expending all that energy healing you.

Curbing your consumption means regularly utilizing your secret weapon with the power of fasting. Research shows that fasting is one of the absolute best things for anti-aging, losing weight, and increasing energy. Fasting is a very simple principle that you can use to put yourself into fat-burning mode quickly.

When you get into a fasting state, you increase your human growth hormone, burn up the excess glucose in your body, optimize your insulin levels, and crank up your metabolism. It helps repair leaky gut by allowing downtime from food digestion so that your body can repair itself.

HOW TO DO INTERMITTENT FASTING

To Implement a fasting regimen focus on periods of time of driving your body into fat-burning mode. If you are a carb addict, or even eat a moderate amount of sugar as we have discussed, you're in sugar- burning mode. If you eat carbohydrates with fat and protein, you're in sugar-burning mode. If you just eat protein, your body converts them to sugar and you're still in sugar-burning mode, although less than from eating straight carbohydrates.

If you eat fat, you can still be a little into sugar-burning mode, but much less than other foods. By using fasting, eating fats and vegetables for your primary fuel, and restricting carbohydrates, you get into fat-burning mode. Adding in high intensity, short duration exercise on top of that will drive you even deeper into fat burning mode.

Fasting is essentially a metabolic workout for your insides, like hitting the gym is a workout for the muscles on the outside. Fasting is the ultimate workout to get your metabolism in shape. Following is how a simple regimen works.

It's a type of scheduled eating plan where you simply restrict your normal daily eating to six to eight hours of time without cutting calories, meaning you're only eating two times during the six to eight-hour window. You can still enjoy a lot of the foods that you love, but you're just allowing your body time to properly digest and then heal.

Care about nutrients during your 6-hour eating window with lots of vegetables and greens. Healthy fats are a must like a coconut oil and avocados. Clean protein will optimize your lean muscle production due to fasting increasing your growth hormone, both male and female.

Not much snacking is needed if you are eating a healthy lunch and a healthy dinner; although if you are hungry in between those two meals in your 6-hour eating window, then raw nuts, an avocado, boiled egg, or low-glycemic fruit like granny smith apples, berries, or grapefruit are a good choice. As with any real-food approach, you want to avoid white bread, pasta, potatoes, starches, and all the processed foods that we've broken down in the previous chapters.

The schedule looks like this. Break. Fast. The first meal of your day is when you break your fast of not eating while you sleep. All you are doing is sliding back that meal and extending the fast. Once you wake up, you skip breakfast. Water, coffee, tea, low-glycemic greens powder, or celery juice could be used to replace breakfast.

Allow your body to stay in the fasting state; so, from waking until 12:00 pm do not consume food or anything that will spike your insulin level. This means you will be in fat-burning mode a lot longer. When you first try this, you may be a little bit hungry, which makes sense if you are used to spiking your insulin and being a sugar-burner all day. Science shows that you have increased energy due to more alertness and minimized sugar crashes due to the restriction of carbohydrate loading.

From 12:00 pm to 6:00 pm you can eat. At first you could eat whatever you'd like. Ideally, you would follow the Make Food Simple guidelines and eliminate snacking. After your 6-hour eating window is over, then it is no food for the next 18 hours. Let your body digest, rest, heal, and crank up the fat-burning. No late night snacks or anything that will spike your insulin. Drink plenty of water and fluids, get extra sleep, and start all over again the next day.

By only eating during a six-hour window, you're giving your body 18 hours to process the food and heal. Your hormones like insulin will be able to store proper energy. Your body

INTERMITTENT FASTING SCHEDULE

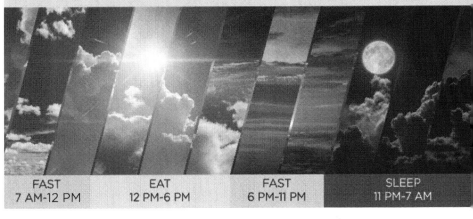

FAST	EAT	FAST	SLEEP
7 AM-12 PM	12 PM-6 PM	6 PM-11 PM	11 PM-7 AM

will hear leptin, and you'll finally burn fat, and grhelin, your hunger hormone, will shut off your appetite. This is what breaks the food addiction and repairs a broken metabolism. Your body mass index (BMI) and weight will normalize, which radically lowers your risk of chronic diseases like diabetes, heart disease, and cancer.

Inflammation will decrease. This is going to lower triglyceride, cholesterol levels, and your risk of heart disease. When your filters have time to heal, instead of digesting food, the free radicals decrease in your body, and you detox. As you detox, you slow down the aging process. When fasting is paired with the principles taught in this book, you will see a rapid acceleration of results. That is what makes curbing your consumption your secret weapon.

MAKE HEALTH SIMPLE

Our forks, knives, spoons, plates, and cups are killing us as a country. We have the ability to take back our health, and it's easier than you think. You may have really messed up your nutrition and your family's. Just respond.
Start practicing the five C's of nutrition. Cut out the sugar and crank up the good fat to balance your hormones and become a fat burner. Clean up the toxicity and reduce your

inflammation. Care about getting nutrients in your system and start making healthy meals at home. Finally, curb your consumption, repair your metabolism, and allow your body to heal. You can do this. You can make food simple. We're here to help, and we're living it along with you. Enjoy the delicious recipes straight from our kitchen to yours and know that you're not alone in this battle to experience real health.

Recipes and meal planning are wonderful when you get the time to actually do them! If you're anything like our family, there are more times than not that we are more "grazing" in our kitchen than actually making 3 full meals a day. Plus, I know myself and my kids rarely need to eat 3 meals a day plus a snack or two (and we aren't starving!).

I am thankful that my kids will eat almost anything I put in front of them; however, I wanted to give you a realistic look at what typical meals and foods look like for them. Because, no, I do not make them these full recipes for every meal. This is just a quick list of things that I always keep on hand and ready each week. If we don't buy anything else--guess what--they don't eat anything else!

Keep Food Simple!
Jessica

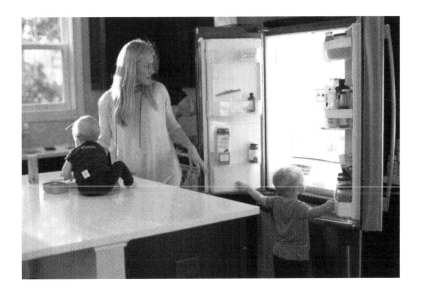

A MESSAGE FROM DR. LIVINGOOD:

Welcome to our kitchen! We are NOT cooks and have no culinary experience to be making a cookbook except this one--we value our health. It's the most important asset we have. This drives our family to eat healthily and figure it out. In order to do that, it has to be simple! We want to let you in--full disclosure to see how we do it. We practice what we preach and preach what we practice. What, your doctor has never shown you his/her kitchen before?

4 THINGS

First I wanted to show you what you would see if you walked in to our kitchen right now, opened a cupboard, fridge, or pantry. That's list one.

Second, Jessica made the comprehensive list of how we feed 3 toddlers every day without processed foods and sugar. None of them have ever needed a drug or hospital visit and are almost too healthy! They wear us out with their healthy energy!

Third, I went one step further and made a comprehensive list of all the approved foods I discussed in chapters one through six. Which foods you can have on the Challenge Plan and which you can have on the Everyday Plan. This serves as a simple eat this--don't eat this list. Use the Challenge Plan until you hit your goals and then stay that way, like my kids, with Everyday Plan foods. As a bonus I also included a food list if you are following an anti-inflammatory plan.

Fourth, in the following recipes, you will find three symbols to help you identify recipes that work on most, if not all, diet plans. The main focus is real food and every recipe in this book can be enjoyed on the Everyday Plan. However, there are specific plans needed at specific times for conditions to heal.

I wanted to allow Jessica and the mommas on our team to make recipes that were easy and delicious. As the doctor, I came behind them and categorized each recipe and gave my alternatives and tips to make recipes work and be approved for specific diets. The last thing I wanted this to do was to make things complicated, so here is my message: You and your kids are safe to enjoy any of these meals made from real food. If you have a specific diet or restrictions, here are the symbols and tips to look for on each recipe to "make it work".

 Anti-Inflammatory: This is the main symbol for the GUT RESET-approved meals. I labeled it the Anti-Inflammatory symbol because it works with most anti-inflammatory diet plans. There are A LOT of anti-inflammatory approaches like AIP, candida diets, Whole 30, and more! All change the rules a bit, but for the most part, when you see this symbol it should be safe. If you don't agree, no big deal, make a substitution or move to another recipe.

 Low Carb: This is the main symbol for the CHALLENGE PLAN-approved meals. I labeled it the Low Carb symbol because it works with most low-carb diet plans. There are A LOT of low carb approaches like keto, paleo, Adkins, South Beach, and more! All change the rules a bit, but for the most part, when you see this symbol it should be safe. If you don't agree, no big deal, make a substitution or move to another recipe. The point is, get as much sugar out as you can, use smart sugar alternatives, and don't stress too much!

 Vegetarian: This is the main symbol for VEGETARIAN approved meals. This does not follow a vegan plan, but follows a vegetarian plan. By definition vegetarians can still have eggs or dairy, but, if you choose not to, then disregard these tips. We made a big effort to make sure you are able to enjoy lots of these recipes even if you don't eat meat or meat products.

The tips and categorization of the recipes bring a ton of flexibility to this cookbook, but I would rather see you keep food simple and actually do it than stress too much and fail.

You have all the tools to Make Food Simple in your hand. Now put them to work to experience real health.

Live Good!
Dr. Livingood

If you go into our kitchen right now, here is what you will find. All of these are found at local stores, health foods stores, Costco, online at Thrive Market or livingooddaily.com through our Livingood Daily Market.

Spices and Oils

All spices are non-irradiated, non-GMO, and organic when possible.

> Sea Salt - Celtic or Himalayan (We use Real Salt brand)
> Pepper
> Garlic Powder
> Cumin
> Chili Powder
> Cinnamon Powder
> Organic Extra Virgin Olive Oil
> Avocado Oil
> Organic Unrefined, Cold-Pressed Coconut Oil
> Organic Apple Cider Vinegar With the Mother
> (Floaters with probiotics and nutrients)
> Natural or Organic Balsamic Vinegar

Baking

All ingredients should be organic when available and free of additives.

> Bread - Organic, Sprouted, Whole Grain, Seeded
> (We use Dave's Killer bread - be sure to check oil)
> Almond Flour
> Coconut Flour
> Tapioca Flour or Arrowroot Powder
> Rolled Oats (Sprouted)
> Chia Seeds, Flax Seeds, and Flax Meal
> Cocoa Powder (Unsweetened)
> Cacao Nibs - Organic and/or No Other Ingredients
> Stevia-Flavored Chocolate Chips
> (We use Lily's brand)
> Baking Soda
> Aluminum-Free Baking Powder
> Organic Pure Vanilla Extract - Ideally Alcohol-Free

Sweeteners

Approved low-glycemic sweeteners are stevia, sugar alcohols (erythritol, xylitol, mannitol, etc), and monk fruit. Natural sweeteners can be used on an everyday plan, but should be restricted on the low-carb challenge plan.

Stevia - Organic, Powdered, and Only Containing Stevia
Swerve Granulated Sugar (Also makes
confectioners sugar and brown sugar)
Organic Coconut Sugar
Organic Maple Syrup - Ideally Grade A, Dark Color
Raw or Organic Local Honey
Monk Fruit

Condiments or Canned Items

Organic Coconut Milk - Full-Fat, Unsweetened, In
BPA-Free Cans or Minimal Ingredient Cartons
Natural or Organic Almond Milk-Unsweetened,
Minimal Ingredient Cartons
Olives - No Additives
Pickles - Water, Salt, Vinegar, and/or Natural Spices
Organic Ketchup - No Sugar Added
Mayonnaise - No Bad Oil (We get Veganaise or
Primal Kitchen brand)
Bragg's Liquid Aminos - Soy Sauce Alternative
Coconut Aminos - Teriyaki Alternative
Nut Butters - Organic, Natural, No Bad Oils Or Sugar

Snacks, Drinks, Other

Coffee - Shade Grown, Organic, and Unflavored
Sparkling Water - No Sugar or Additives (We love Spindrift)
Nuts - Raw or Dry Roasted (We get Costco or
Trader Joe's brand)
Chips - Cassava Root Based (We get Siete brand)
Crackers - Only Approved Fours and No Bad Oils (We use
Simple Mills brand)
Berries - Fresh and Frozen, Wild, and Ideally Organic
Fruit - Granny Smith Apples and Oranges
Veggies - Broccoli, Cucumbers, Purple Cabbage and
Spinach
Roots - Sweet Potatoes
Hummus - No Bad Oils, Organic
Eggs - Organic, Free-Range
Meat - Boiled Organic Free Range Chicken

Breakfast

Smoothies
Mixed berries (+ occasional ½ organic banana)
Scrambled eggs
Egg Bake
Turkey bacon
Organic turkey sausage
Grass-fed yogurt with Livingood Daily Collagen
        mixed in and berries (occasional)

Lunch

Cooked chicken dipped in hummus (we always keep
        cooked chicken in the fridge)
Raw veggies dipped in hummus (we always keep
        cut-up veggies in a large container)
Raw organic cheese chunks
Leftover sweet potato chunks from dinner (or any
        leftover for that matter)
Turkey roll-ups (with hummus inside)

Dinner

Hamburger (no bun) dipped in ketchup
Simple sautéed sweet potatoes or sweet potato
        fries
Veggies dipped in hummus
Roasted broccoli and brussel sprouts
Chicken and hummus
Grass-fed hotdogs (occasionally)
Chicken and black bean quesadillas with raw cheese
        and Siete or spelt wraps (occasionally)
Smoothie Bowls

Sides & Snacks

Black olives
Black beans (yes, they will eat them out of the jar)
Raw organic cheese
Veggies and hummus
Fruit (berries, oranges, organic grapes, dried fruit,
        etc)
Apple slices with almond butter
Livingood Daily Chocolate Bars (careful, they will
        become hooked)
Nuts – any kind of nuts
Livingood Daily Goods Bars
Pickles
Simple Mills Crackers or Siete Chips (Occassionally)

Drinks

Water!
Livingood Daily Greens (would drink this all day if
        we let them)
"Spicy water" (what our kids call sparkling water +
        we always add Livingood Daily High Dose
        Vitamin C Powder)
Smoothies (they love any flavor)
"Chocolate milk" (Livingood Daily Collagen
        Chocolate or Livingood Daily Greens
        Chocolate in coconut or almond milk)

FOOD LIST

MEATS

- [ ] Beef / Buffalo / Venison
  Ideally All Natural, Best is 100% Grass-Fed & Organic
- [ ] Chicken
  Ideally All Natural, Best is Organic & Free Range
- [ ] Eggs
  Ideally All Natural, Best is Organic & Free Range
- [ ] Fish: Wild Caught

- [ ] Lamb
  Ideally All Natural, Best is 100% Grass-Fed & Organic
- [ ] Turkey
  Ideally All Natural, Best is Organic & Free Range

Avoid
Grain-Fed, Pork, Farm-Raised Fish, Shellfish, and Soy Alternatives

VEGETABLES

[ ] Arugula	[ ] Cucumbers	[ ] Onions	**In Moderation**
[ ] Asparagus	[ ] Dandelion	[ ] Parsley	[ ] Artichokes
[ ] Beans	[ ] Eggplant	[ ] Radishes	[ ] Beets
[ ] Bell Peppers	[ ] Fennel	[ ] Shallots	[ ] Carrots
[ ] Bok Coy	[ ] Garlic	[ ] Snow Peas	[ ] Jicama
[ ] Broccoli	[ ] Green Beans	[ ] Spinach	[ ] Squash
[ ] Brussels Sprouts	[ ] Jalapeno Peppers	[ ] Sprouts	[ ] Sweet Potatoes
[ ] Cabbage	[ ] Kale	[ ] Turnips	[ ] Tomatoes
[ ] Cauliflower	[ ] Kohlrabi	[ ] Water Chestnuts	**Avoid**
[ ] Celery	[ ] Lettuce	[ ] Zucchini	Corn
[ ] Chicory	[ ] Mushrooms		Potatoes
[ ] Collard	[ ] Mustard		

FRUITS

Ideally All Natural, Best is Organic

[ ] Acai Berries	[ ] Grapefruit
[ ] Avocado	[ ] Lemon
[ ] Blackberries	[ ] Lime
[ ] Granny Smith Apples	[ ] Raspberries
[ ] Blueberries	[ ] Strawberries

Avoid Until Goal Is Hit

[ ] Apricots	[ ] Oranges
[ ] Bananas	[ ] Papaya
[ ] Cherries	[ ] Peaches
[ ] Dates	[ ] Pears
[ ] Grapes	[ ] Pineapple
[ ] Kiwi	[ ] Plum
[ ] Mangoes	[ ] Prunes
[ ] Melon	[ ] Red Apples
[ ] Nectarines	[ ] Dried Fruit
[ ] Watermelon	[ ] Goji Berries

DAIRY

Ideally All Natural, Best is Organic, Full Fat, & Raw - In Moderation

[ ] Butter	[ ] Organic Milk	
[ ] Cheese	[ ] Almond Milk	**Avoid**
[ ] Cream	[ ] Cashew Milk	Margarine
[ ] Goat's Milk	[ ] Coconut Milk	Shortening
[ ] Goat's Milk Cheese	[ ] Goat Milk	Soy
[ ] Goat's Milk Yogurt	[ ] Hemp Milk	Non-Organic Dairy
[ ] Kefir	[ ] Ghee	

FOOD LIST

Best is Raw, Organic and/or Sprouted With No Added Oils
In Moderation

- [ ] Almonds
- [ ] Brazil
- [ ] Cashews
- [ ] Chia Seeds
- [ ] Flax Seeds
- [ ] Hemp Seeds
- [ ] Macadamia

- [ ] Pecans
- [ ] Pine Nuts
- [ ] Pistachios
- [ ] Pumpkin Seeds
- [ ] Sesame Seeds
- [ ] Sunflower Seeds
- [ ] Walnuts

- [ ] Almond Butter
- [ ] Cashew Butter
- [ ] Macadamia Butter
- [ ] Sunflower Seed Butter
- [ ] Tahini (Raw)
- [ ] Valencia Peanut Butter

Avoid / Limit
Peanut Butter
(Non-Valencia)

Ideally All Natural, Best is Unrefined & Cold-Pressed

- [ ] Avocado Oil
- [ ] Butter/Ghee (Low Heat)
- [ ] Coconut Oil
- [ ] Flaxseed Oil (Do Not Heat)
- [ ] Grapeseed Oil
- [ ] Olive Oil (Medium/Low Heat)

Avoid
Canola Oil
Corn Oil
Cotton Seed Oil
Rapeseed Oil
Rice Bran Oil
Safflower Oil
Soybean Oil
Sunflower Oil
Vegetable Oil

In Moderation

- [ ] Adzuki Beans
- [ ] Black Beans
- [ ] Chickpeas
- [ ] Kidney Beans
- [ ] Legumes

- [ ] Lentils
- [ ] Lima Beans
- [ ] Pinto Beans
- [ ] White Beans

- [ ] Allulose
- [ ] 100% Stevia
- [ ] Xylitol (In Moderation)
- [ ] Monk Fruit
- [ ] Erythritol

Avoid Until Goal Is Hit
- [ ] Raw Honey
- [ ] Organic Maple Syrup (Grade A/B)

Avoid
All Added Sugars
Aspartame
Dextrose
Fructose
Glucose
Maltodextrin
Splenda
Sucrose
Artificial Sweetners

Avoid Until Goal Is Hit

- [ ] Barley
- [ ] Brown/Wild Rice
- [ ] Buckwheat
- [ ] Ezekiel 4:9 Bread
- [ ] Millet
- [ ] Quinoa

- [ ] Rye
- [ ] Spelt
- [ ] Steel Cut Oats
- [ ] Tapioca
- [ ] Sprouted Grain Bread
- [ ] Whole/Wild Grains

Best is Unsweetened, Raw or Organic With No Added Sugars | Sweeten with Stevia
In Moderation

- [ ] Coffee
- [ ] Herbal Tea
- [ ] Water (Infused, Purified, And/Or Sparkling)
- [ ] Low Sugar Fruit/Vegetable Juice

Avoid Until Goal Is Hit
- [ ] Fermented Drinks
- [ ] Fruit/Vegetable Juice
- [ ] Coconut Water
- [ ] Zevia/Stevia Sweetened Soda

Best is All Natural or Organic

- [ ] Apple Cider Vinegar
- [ ] Balsamic Vinegar
- [ ] Guacamole
- [ ] Herbs/Spices
- [ ] Hummus (No Bad Oil)
- [ ] Mustard
- [ ] Olive Oil

- [ ] Salsa
- [ ] Sea Salt (Celtic or Himalayan)
- [ ] Soy Sauce (Liquid Aminos, Wheat Free)
- [ ] Mayo (Veganaise or Avocado-Oil Based)

Anti-Inflammatory Food
To Avoid List

AVOID THESE COMPLETELY

Proceed With Caution

*If you know you have a sensitivity, avoid these foods. If you are not sensitive or are unsure, consume in moderation. (1-2 times per week)

Pantry

Coconut Milk
Coconut Oil
Coconut Flakes
Coconut Flour
Chia Seeds
Cous Cous
Coffee
Dark Chocolate >70%
Cacao >70%
Flaxseed
Gogi Berries
Guinoa
Tomatoes

Beans & Legumes

Adzuki Beans
Black Beans
Black Eyed Peas
Chickpeas
Fava Beans
Kidney Bean
Lentils
Lima Beans
Peanuts
Soybeans

Nuts

Almond
Brazil
Cashews
Cocoa
Hazelnut
Pecan
Macadamia
Pistashios
Walnut

Grains

Amaranth
Barley
Buckwheat
Bulgur
Corn
Farro
Kamut
Millet
Oats
Rice
Rye
Sorghum
Spelt
Teff
Wheat

Dairy

Butter
Cheese
Cream
Cream Cheese
Ghee
Milk
Yogurt

Alcohol

Beer
Champagne
Hard Cider
Liquor
Malt Beverages
Wine

Eggs

Chicken
Duck
Egg White
Egg Yolk
Quail
Goose

Nightshades

Bell Pepper
Black Pepper
Cayenne
Chili Pepper
Chipotle
Eggplant
Habanero
Jalepeno
Paprika
Poblano
Red Pepper
Sweet Pepper
Tobacco
Tomatillo
White Potato

Seeds

Anise
Canola
Caraway
Coriander
Cumin
Fennel
Fennugreek
Hemp
Mustard
Nutmeg
Poppy
Pumpkin
Sesame
Sunflower

NSAIDS

Asprin
Ibuprofen

Anti-Inflammatory Food List

Vegetables

Artichoke
Asparagus
Bok Choy
Broccoli
Brussels Sprouts
Cabbage
Cauliflower
Celery
Chard
Collard Greens
Cucumber
Fennel
Green Beans
Kale
Leek
Lettuce
Mushroom
Spinach
Squash
Watercress
Zucchini

Pantry Items

Apple Cider Vinegar
Arrowroot Powder
Arrowroot Flour
Canned Fish
Coconut Vinegar
Coconut Sugar
Coconut Aminos
Dried Fruit
Honey
Maple Syrup
Olives
Palm Sugar

Fats

Animal Fat
Avocado Oil
Coconut Butter
Lard
Olive Oil
Palm Oil
Tallow

Herbs & Spices

Basil
Chives
Cilantro
Cinnamon
Cloves
Dill
Garlic
Ginger
Lemongrass
Marjoram
Mint
Parsley
Rosemary
Saffron
Sage
Sea Salt
Shallots
Thyme
Turmeric

Roots

Beets
Carrots
Celeriac
Jicama
Maca
Onion
Parsnip
Turnip
Radish
Rutabaga
Shallot
Sweet Potato
Yam

Meats

Beef
Bison
Buffalo
Chicken
Duck
Elk
Fish
Lamb
Turkey
Venison

Offal

Bone Broth
Heart
Kidney
Liver
Sardines

Fruits

Apple
Apricot
Avocado
Banana
Blackberries
Blueberries
Cherry
Clementine
Coconut
Cranberries
Date
Fig
Grape
Grapefruit
Kiwi
Lemon
Lime
Mango
Melon
Nectarine
Orange
Papaya
Peach
Pear
Plum
Pineapple
Pomegranate
Stawberries
Tangerine

Fermented

Fermented Veggies
(Carrot, Beet, ect.)
Kombucha
Meso
Natto
Olives
Pickles
Sauerkraut
Tamari
Tempeh
Water Kefir

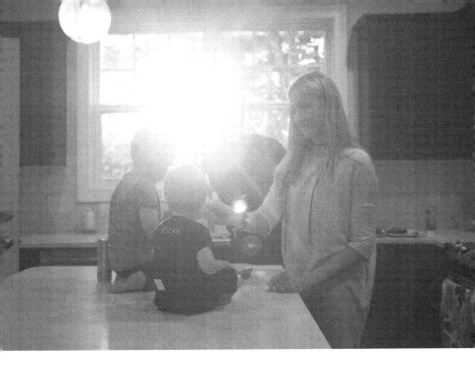

From Our Kitchen To Yours

I am a wife, a mom of three kiddos--all 4 and under--and I also work full time, plus some! Oh, and I love to eat! I'd call myself a foodie, but that sounds too fancy for what I eat! Let's be honest--I have little time left in a day to cook fancy meals, using a ton of ingredients that I have to prep, and having left over ingredients that will just go to waste after one recipe. I need simple. Very simple and fast! These recipes might not be extravagant or things you haven't thought of or made before. However, if you're like me, you need quick and easy meal IDEAS that are also healthy and nutritious. Here are some of my family's quick and easy, and in our opinion, delicious recipes. Oh, did I mention time? Speaking of, I don't usually have time to measure either. That being said, most of these recipes are my best guess, so feel free to tweak them to your own liking. ;)

Keep Food Simple,
Jessica Livingood

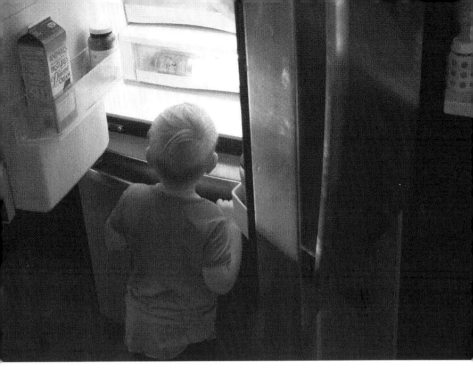

TABLE OF CONTENTS

Breakfast   89

Smoothies   103

Main Dishes   111

Side Dishes   143

Salads + Soups   155

Desserts   169

Drinks   183

Snacks   195

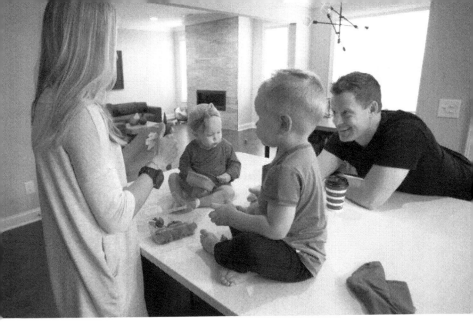

BREAKFAST

DLG Donuts   90

Egg Scramble   92

Simple Muffin Batter   93

Egg in Avocado   94

Blueberry Lemon Scones   95

On-The-Go Eggs   96

DLG Cereal   97

DLG Anti-Inflammatory Porridge   98

Simple Pancakes   99

DLG Overnight Oats   100

Chipotle Avocado Toast   101

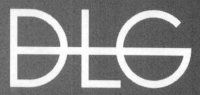

DLG Donuts

Serves 6 | 25 Minutes

Donuts:
1 tbsp butter (to grease pan)

1 1/2 cups almond flour

3 organic eggs (*see next page for the egg-free substitute)

3 tsp vanilla extract

1/2 tsp baking soda

2 tbsp honey

Topping:
4 tbsp butter (melted)

3 tbsp Swerve sweetener or coconut sugar

1 tbsp cinnamon (to taste)

Donuts:
In a bowl, mix all ingredients together until smooth. Grease donut pan and fill until approximately 3/4 full. Bake at 300 degrees F for approximately 10-15 minutes or until slightly light brown on top - keep a close eye on them. Do not let them overcook or they will be dry. Allow to cool for 5 minutes before taking them out of the donut pan.

Topping:
Melt the butter and set aside. Mix the sugar substitute and cinnamon in a bowl. Dip the top of the donut into the butter, just enough to coat the top. Then dip the top of the donut into the sugar mixture. I recommend eating these donuts while they are still slightly warm for the best taste! If you choose to leave some for the next day or two, I would wait to top/coat the donuts until you are ready to eat them.

I prefer the cinnamon and "sugar" topping but some love a good frosting on top! Try the frosting recipe on the next page!

Low Carb Plan Tip:
Remove the sweetener (honey/maple syrup) and try coconut sugar, xylitol, or stevia, to taste.

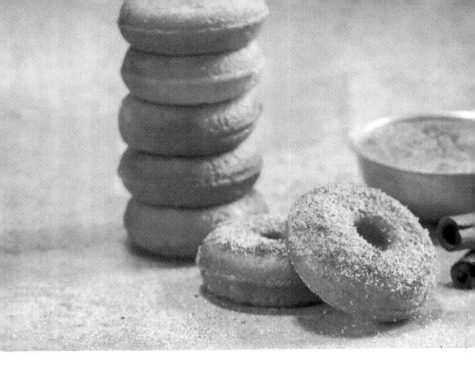

DLG Donuts

Continued From Previous Page

Flax Egg | Egg-Free Substitution:
Grind 3 tbsp of flax seeds in a coffee grinder (can buy pre-ground also) Mix 3 tbsp ground flax seeds with 9 tbsp water. Stir and let sit in the fridge for approximately 30 minutes. Use these flax eggs instead of eggs!

Optional Frosting Topping:
Slowly melt the coconut butter on low heat. Remove from the heat and add vanilla and sweetener. Add the milk one tablespoon at a time, stirring in between until a smooth, frosting-like consistency.

Anti-Inflammatory Plan Tip:
Instead of eggs, follow the flax egg option. Replace the butter with coconut or avocado oil.

Vegetarian Plan Tip:
Approved for vegetarians that eat eggs and/or dairy.

Flax Eggs:
3 tbsp flax seeds (ground up)

9 tbsp water

Optional Frosting Topping:
6 tbsp coconut butter (melted)

1 tsp vanilla extract

2 tbsp Swerve Confectioners' Sweetener

4-6 tbsp unsweetened almond milk (or other non-dairy milk of choice) until thin and frosting-like

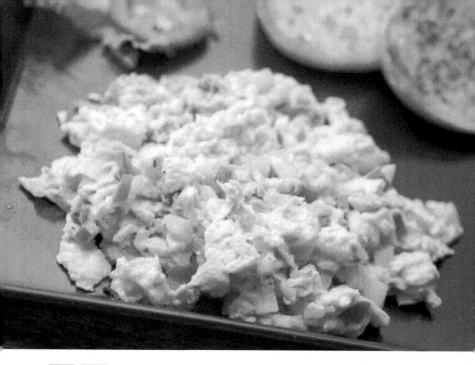

Egg Scramble

Serves 2 | 15 Minutes

4 organic eggs

1 cup vegetables (diced) - any combination of bell peppers, spinach, zucchini, mushrooms, broccoli, onion, etc. - or whatever vegetables you have on hard

1/2 cup turkey bacon or turkey sausage (pre-cooked) (optional)

Salt and pepper (to taste)

2 tbsp coconut oil

Optional toppings: avocado, organic cheese (cheddar, feta, goat, etc), chives

Whisk eggs, veggies, pre-cooked meat, if adding, and seasonings in a bowl. In medium pan, heat oil over medium/low heat. Cook and scramble for 6-8 minutes until eggs are cooked through. Top with favorite toppings.

Vegetarian Plan Tip:
Approved for vegetarians that eat eggs and/or dairy.

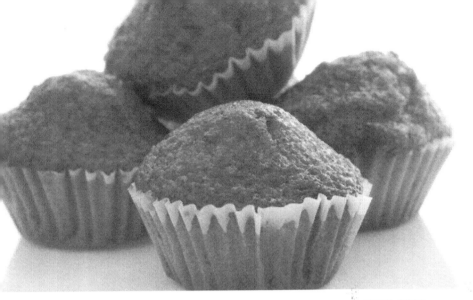

Simple Muffin Batter

Yields 8-10 Muffins | 20 Minutes

In a mixing bowl, stir together the eggs, coconut oil, apple cider vinegar, vanilla extract, and honey. Once combined, add the almond four, baking soda and sea salt. Mix well and add your flavor of choice. Spoon the batter into muffin tins lightly greased with coconut oil. Bake at 350 degrees F for approximately 20 minutes or until golden brown and cooked through.

Low Carb Plan Tip:
Remove the sweetener (honey/maple syrup) and try coconut sugar, xylitol, or stevia, to taste.

Vegetarian Plan Tip:
Approved for vegetarians that eat eggs and/or dairy.

3 organic eggs

4 tbsp coconut oil or butter (melted) + 1 tsp to grease pan

1 tbsp apple cider vinegar

2 tsp vanilla extract

2 tbsp honey

2 cups almond flour

1/2 tsp baking soda

1/2 tsp sea salt

Optional flavor add-ins:
Berry: 1 cup fresh or frozen berries of choice

Banana nut: 1 less egg, 2 ripe bananas, & chopped walnuts

Cinnamon: 1 1/2 tsp cinnamon

Chocolate chip: 1/2 cup stevia-sweetened chocolate chips

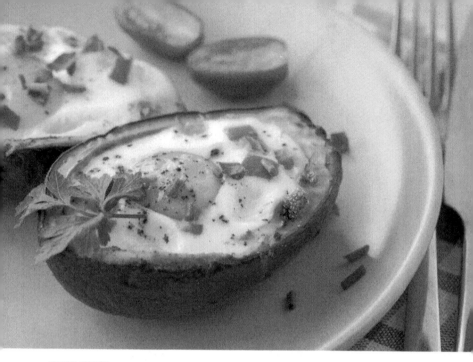

Egg In Avocado

Serves 1 | 25 Minutes

1 avocado

2 organic eggs

Salt and pepper (to taste)

Optional: top with turkey bacon (pre-cooked) and/or chives

Slice the avocado in half and remove the pit. Place in a small baking dish. Crack an egg into each avocado half. Bake at 425 degrees F for approximately 15-20 minutes. Remove and add salt, pepper, pre-cooked turkey bacon, and/or chives, if desired.

Vegetarian Plan Tip:
Approved for vegetarians that eat eggs and/or dairy.

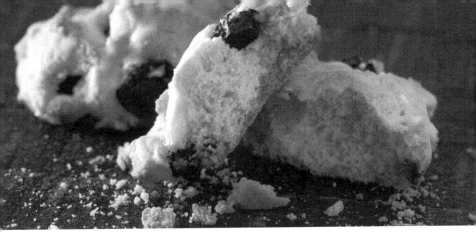

Blueberry Lemon Scones

Yields 8 Scones | 45 Minutes

In a food processor, combine the almond flour, baking soda and sea salt. Pulse in the cold butter until the butter is approximately pea-sized. In a large bowl, whisk the eggs, coconut milk, lemon zest, lemon juice and the honey until combined. Using a spoon, stir the dry mixture into the wet mixture until thoroughly combined. Fold in the blueberries. Place the dough mix in the fridge to chill for approximately 15 minutes. Once the dough is chilled, roll it into a ball and place it on an almond flour sprinkled surface. Roll out and shape the dough into a square that is approximately 6"x6" and 1" thick. Cut the dough square in half, twice, to make 4 small squares. Then cut each of the small squares in half diagonally to make 8 small triangles. Brush the top with melted butter and sprinkle with coconut sugar, if desired. Bake at 350 degrees F, on a parchment lined baking sheet, for 15 minutes or until slightly golden.

Low Carb Plan Tip:
Remove the sweetener (honey/maple syrup) and try coconut sugar, xylitol, or stevia, to taste.

Vegetarian Plan Tip:
Approved for vegetarians that eat eggs and/or dairy.

2 3/4 cups almond flour

1/2 tsp baking soda

1/4 tsp sea salt

2 tbsp butter (cold)

2 organic eggs

2 tbsp coconut milk

1 tsp lemon zest

2 tsp lemon juice

1 tbsp honey or 5-10 drops of liquid stevia (to taste)

1/3 cup blueberries (fresh, frozen, or dried)

Optional: 2 tbsp butter (melted) and 2 tsp coconut sugar (topping)

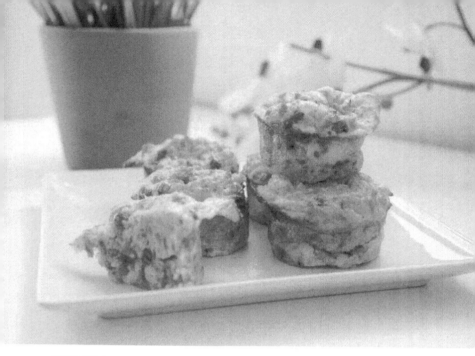

On-The-Go Eggs
Serves 6 | 30 Minutes

1 tsp coconut oil (to grease pan)

8 organic eggs

1 cup vegetables (diced) - any combination of broccoli, peppers, onion, mushrooms, etc. - or whatever vegetables you have on hand

Salt and pepper (to taste)

1/2 cup organic cheese (optional)

1/2 cup turkey bacon (pre-cooked) (optional)

1/2 cup coconut or unsweetened almond milk (optional)

Lightly grease a muffin tin with coconut oil. Whisk eggs, vegetables, optional turkey bacon, and optional coconut/almond milk together. Add salt and pepper. Pour into muffin tins. Bake 350 degrees F for 20-25 minutes.

Vegetarian Plan Tip: Approved for vegetarians that eat eggs and/or dairy.

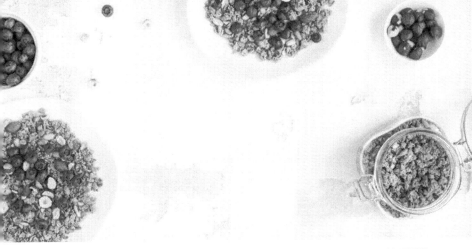

DLG Cereal

Serves 4 | 10-30 Minutes (Depending On If Baking)

Option 1:
Put all nuts, seeds, collagen protein, and cinnamon in a blender and blend until a fine consistency (think Grape Nuts cereal). You will not use the vanilla extract or coconut oil for this recipe.

Option 2: Granola-Like
Stir all ingredients in a bowl until mixed together well. Spread evenly on a parchment paper lined cookie sheet. Bake for approximately 20-30 minutes at 300 degrees F. Be sure to stir frequently to prevent it from burning. Allow to cool completely before serving.

Anti-Inflammatory Plan Tip:
Coconut, almonds, flaxseeds, and other nuts/seeds are options for this plan, in moderation, if no known sensitivities.

Vegetarian Plan Tip:
Approved for vegetarians that eat eggs and/or dairy.

1 cup almonds (slivered)

1/2 cup flax seeds

1/3 cup sunflower seeds

1 cup mix of other nuts or seeds: pepitas, crushed pecans, crushed cashews, crushed, crushed walnuts, etc.

1/2 cup unsweetened coconut flakes (shredded)

2 tbsp cinnamon

1 scoop Livingood Daily Vanilla Collagen Protein

1 tsp vanilla extract (option 2 only)

1/3 cup coconut oil (option 2 only)

Unsweetened almond milk (for serving)

Optional toppings: raisins, berries, unsweetened coconut flakes, Livingood Daily Vanilla Collagen Protein

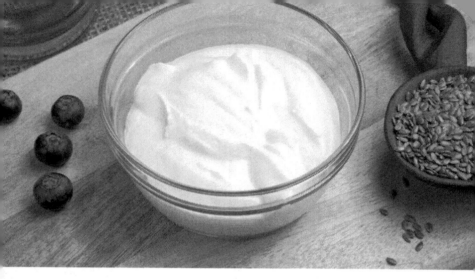

DLG Anti-Inflammatory Porridge

Serves 1 | 15 Minutes

6 tbsp organic cottage cheese (or kefir)

3 tbsp organic flax oil

3 tbsp organic flax seeds (ground up into meal)*

1 tsp turmeric powder (for anti-inflammatory)

Optional toppings:
2 tbsp almond butter

1 tbsp coconut manna or coconut butter

1/2 cup berries of choice

1 tbsp honey

1/2 scoop Livingood Daily Vanilla Collagen Protein

Combine cottage cheese and oil in a bowl and use a hand blender to blend until smooth. Stir in flax meal and turmeric, if using. Top with any of your favorite toppings and enjoy!

This delicious breakfast treat for the whole family is easy to make and super nutritious. Used as a long-standing anti-cancer protocol, the combination of flax seeds, flax seed oil, and the sulfur from the cottage cheese make this a super food for your cells. It acts as a powerful anti-inflammatory to relieve aches, pains, and is good for the gut.

*Do not include flax seed if you have colorectal cancer or a colostomy.

Low Carb Plan Tip:
Remove the sweetener (honey/maple syrup) and use Livingood Daily Vanilla Collagen Protein to sweeten. You can also try coconut sugar, xylitol, or stevia, to taste.

Vegetarian Plan Tip:
Approved for vegetarians that eat eggs and/or dairy.

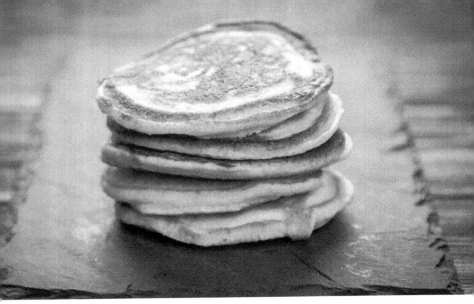

Simple Pancakes

Yields 8 Pancakes | 20 Minutes

Using a high-powered blender (for best results) or a hand held mixer, mix all wet ingredients in a bowl. In a separate bowl, mix all dry ingredients together. Add the wet ingredients to the dry ingredients and mix until smooth. Using an oil-greased pan over medium/low heat, pour the batter into desired sized pancakes. Flip when you start to see little air bubbles, or approximately 2-3 minutes. Cook approximately another 2 minutes.

Low Carb Plan Tip:
Avoid the syrup or honey while on a low carb plan. Try adding some fresh, organic berries to a small pot with a splash of water. Smash berries with a fork and warm the berry/water mixture. Serve over pancakes.

Vegetarian Plan Tip:
Approved for vegetarians that eat eggs and/or dairy.

1/4-1/2 cup unsweetened almond milk

4 large eggs

1 tbsp honey or maple syrup

1 tsp apple cider vinegar

1 tsp vanilla extract

1/2 cup almond flour

1/3 cup tapioca flour

1/4 cup coconut flour

1/2 tsp salt

1 tsp baking soda

1 tbsp butter, olive oil, or coconut oil (for greasing)

1/4 cup of fresh berries (optional)

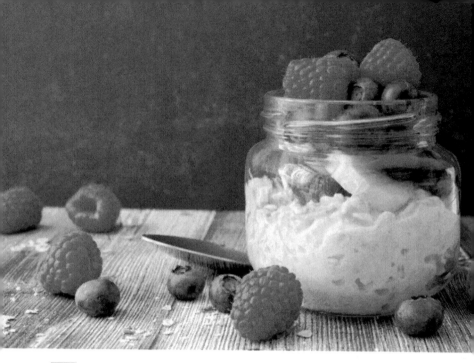

DLG Overnight Oats

Serves 2 | 10 Minutes + 4 Hours Chill Time

1 cup rolled or quick oats

1/2 cup coconut milk

1/2 cup unsweetened almond milk

1 tbsp chia seeds

1 tsp vanilla extract

1/2 tsp sea salt

1 tbsp maple syrup (optional)

1/2 scoop of LIvingood Daily Vanilla Collagen

Optional toppings: coconut flakes, berries, chia seeds

Combine all ingredients and stir until mixed well. Put in the fridge to chill for a minimum of 4 hours (best if overnight).

Low Carb Plan Tip:
Avoid this recipe on a no sugar plan and use the DLG Cereal recipe (page 97) as another option.

Vegetarian Plan Tip:
Approved for vegetarians that eat eggs and/or dairy.

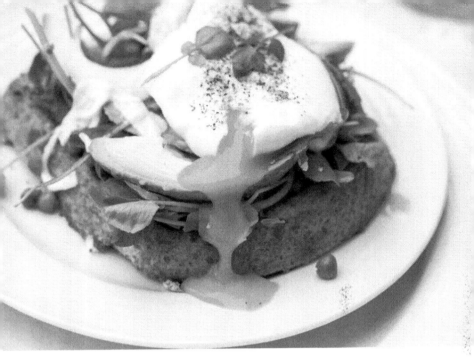

Chipotle Avocado Toast

Serves 1 | 15 Minutes

Fry an egg on medium/low heat in coconut oil. Toast your bread and spread chipotle mayo on it. Sprinkle with the sprouts. Slice the half of avocado and the roma tomato and lay on bread. Place your fried egg on top with pre-cooked turkey bacon, if desired.

Vegetarian Plan Tip:
Approved for vegetarians that eat eggs and/or dairy.

1 organic egg

2 tbsp coconut oil

1 piece of sprouted bread (toasted)

1 tbsp chipotle mayo (I just buy Primal Kitchen brand to avoid bad oils)

1 handful of sprouts

1/2 avocado

1/2 organic roma tomato

Optional topping: turkey bacon (pre-cooked)

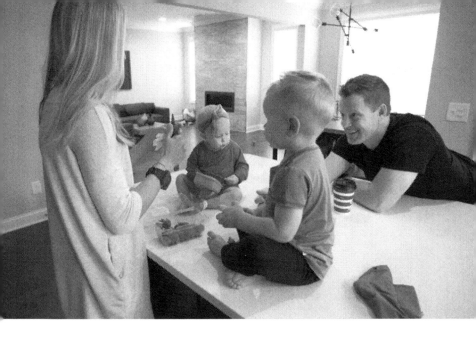

SMOOTHIES

Berry Simple Smoothie   104

Chocolate Almond Smoothie   105

Berry Smoothie Bowl   106

Almond Joy Smoothie   107

DLG Favorite Smoothie   108

The Ultimate Smoothie   109

The Chocolate Coffee Smoothie 110

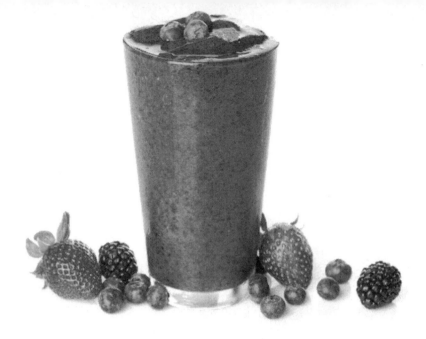

Berry Simple Smoothie

Serves 1 | 10 Minutes

1 cup spinach

1/4-1/2 can coconut milk or unsweetened nut milk

1/2 cup of water (and/or ice to make thicker and colder)

1 cup of frozen berries of choice (if using fresh berries add 4 ice cubes)

1/3 of a frozen banana (optional)

1 scoop Livingood Daily Vanilla Collagen Protein

1/4-1/2 an avocado (cubed then frozen, optional - for a thicker and smoother consistency)

Combine all ingredients in a high-powered blender and mix until smoothie consistency. Use more or less of any ingredient to make thicker, thinner, or colder.

Low Carb Plan Tip:
Skip the 1/3 of a banana.

Vegetarian Plan Tip:
Use a vegetarian protein or Livingood Daily Greens in place of the Collagen Protein.

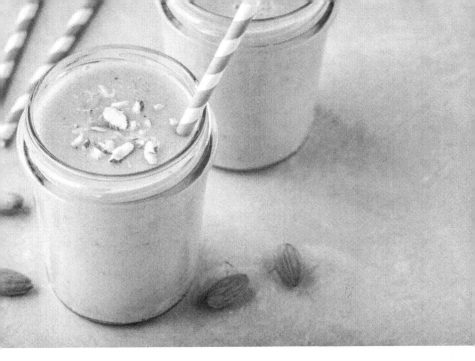

Chocolate Almond Smoothie

Serves 1 | 10 Minutes

Put all ingredients in a blender and mix. Can add more or less nut milk depending on the size of smoothie desired.

Anti-Inflammatory Plan Tip:
Coconut, almond, cashew, and flax milk or butter are options for this plan as well as chocolate, cacao, and coffee, in moderation, if no known sensitivities.

Vegetarian Plan Tip:
Use a vegetarian protein or Livingood Daily Greens in place of the Collagen Protein.

1 scoop Livingood Daily Chocolate Collagen Protein (or 1 tbsp cocoa powder with 1 scoop Livingood Daily Vanilla Collagen Protein)

3 tbsp almond or another nut butter

1/4-1/2 cup unsweetened almond milk or coconut milk

1/4-1/2 an avocado (cubed then frozen, optional - for a thicker and smoother consistency)

3-4 ice cubes (optional)

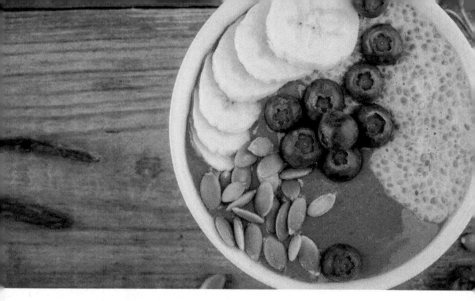

Berry Smoothie Bowl
Serves 1 | 10 Minutes

1/2-1 cup coconut milk

1 1/2 cups frozen berries or fruit of your choice

1/2 frozen banana (optional)

1 scoop Livingood Daily Vanilla Collagen Protein (optional, but yummy)

1 tbsp flax seeds and/or chia seeds

Optional add-Ins but yummy and nutritious: 1 package organic no sugar acai and/or 1 package organic acerola cherry (I use Trader Joe's brands)

Optional toppings: fresh fruit sliced, chia seeds, sliced almonds or nuts, toasted or dried coconut flakes, granola, cacao nibs, stevia-sweetened chocolate chips

Put the coconut milk in a high powered blender first, then add the frozen fruit on top. This is meant to be thick and hard to blend, keep pushing the fruit down into the blender until smooth and thick. If you do need a little more coconut milk you can always add a little more. Add the half scoop of collagen at the end and blend together. Pour the smoothie into a bowl and top with your favorite toppings.

Anti-Inflammatory Plan Tip: Coconut, almond, cashew, and flax milk or butter are options for this plan as well as chocolate, cacao, and coffee, in moderation, if no known sensitivities.

Low Carb Plan Tip: Stick to berries only. Sub the half of a banana option with a few chunks of frozen avocado for extra fat.

Vegetarian Plan Tip: Use a vegetarian protein or Livingood Daily Greens in place of the Collagen Protein.

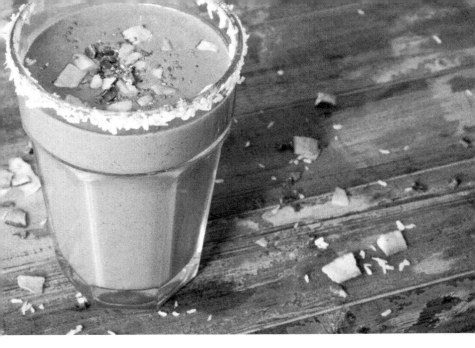

Almond Joy Smoothie

Serves 1 | 10 Minutes

Put all ingredients into a high powered blender and blend until smooth. Can give or take amounts of smoothie ingredients to your liking! This smoothie is so good it could be a snack, drink, or dessert!

Anti-Inflammatory Plan Tip: Coconut, almond, cashew, and flax milk or butter are options for this plan as well as chocolate, cacao, and coffee, in moderation, if no known sensitivities.

Low Carb Plan Tip: Avoid bananas during a low carb plan. Opt for a few chunks of frozen avocado instead.

Vegetarian Plan Tip: Use a vegetarian protein or Livingood Daily Greens in place of the Collagen Protein.

1/4-1/2 cup unsweetened almond milk

1/2 frozen banana

2 large spoon fulls of almond butter

1 tbsp cocoa powder

1 tsp cinnamon

1 tsp vanilla extract

1/2 scoop Livingood Daily Chocolate Collagen Protein

1/4-1/2 an avocado (cubed then frozen) (optional)

Optional topping: shredded coconut (unsweetened)

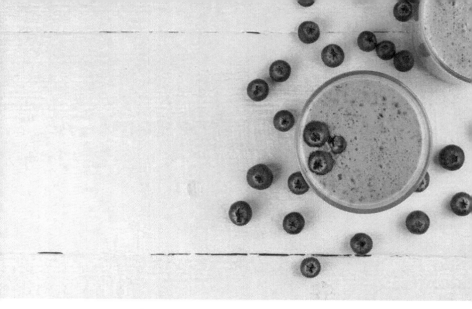

DLG Favorite Smoothie
Serves 1 | 10 Minutes

1 large handful of spinach

1/4-1/2 cup coconut milk or unsweetened almond milk

1/2-3/4 cup frozen blueberries

2 large spoon fulls of almond butter

1 scoop Livingood Daily Vanilla Collagen Protein

Cacao nibs (optional)

Flax and/or chia seeds (optional)

3-4 ice cubes (optional)

Put all ingredients in a blender and mix. Can add more or less nut milk depending on the size of smoothie desired.

Anti-Inflammatory Plan Tip: Coconut, almond, cashew, and flax milk or butter are options for this plan as well as chocolate, cacao, and coffee, in moderation, if no known sensitivities.

Vegetarian Plan Tip: Use a vegetarian protein or Livingood Daily Greens in place of the Collagen Protein.

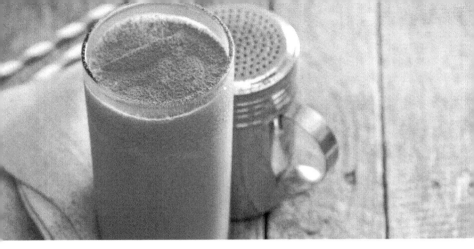

The Ultimate Smoothie

Serves 1 | 10 Minutes

Put all ingredients except protein powder into a blender. Blend until smooth. Add protein powder and blend on low speed until it is all mixed in. Add more or less liquid to desired consistency and more or less ice to desired temperature.

Vegetarian Plan Tip:
Use a vegetarian protein or Livingood Daily Greens in place of the Collagen Protein.

1/4-1/2 cup coconut milk

1/4 cup unsweetened, vanilla almond milk

1 cup of spinach

1 tbsp cocoa powder (especially if you do not add chocolate protein)

2 tbsp cacao nibs

2 tbsp whole flax seeds

2 tbsp chia seeds

1 tbsp maca root powder

1 scoop Livingood Daily Greens Powder (optional but yummy!)

1 tbsp coconut oil

1/2 cup water or nut milk (for desired smoothie consistency)

3-4 ice cubes

1 scoop of Livingood Daily Collagen Protein (try 1/2 vanilla 1/2 chocolate)

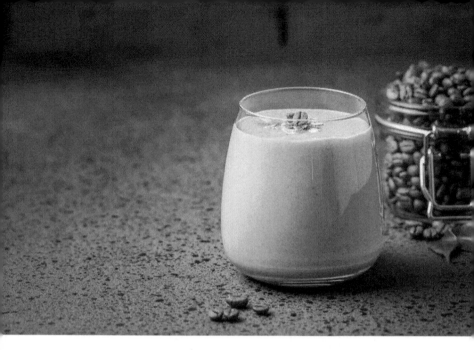

 ## The Chocolate Coffee Smoothie

Serves 1 | 15 Minutes

1/2 cup of brewed organic coffee (cooled to room temperature)

1/4-1/2 cup coconut milk or 1/2 cup unsweetened nut milk

2 tbsp almond butter

1 tsp cinnamon powder

1 tsp cacao

1/2 frozen banana (optional)

3-4 ice cubes

1/2 scoop Livingood Daily Chocolate Collagen Protein (optional but yummy!)

1 tbsp maca root powder (optional)

Put all ingredients except protein powder into a blender. Blend until smooth. Add protein powder and blend on low speed until it is all mixed in. Add more or less liquid to desired consistency and more or less ice to desired temperature.

Low Carb Plan Tip:
Skip the banana
(but you won't miss it!)

Vegetarian Plan Tip:
Use a vegetarian protein or Livingood Daily Greens in place of the Collagen Protein.

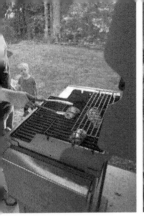
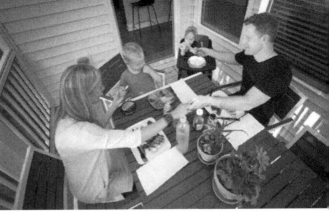

MAIN DISHES

DLG Casserole — 112
Slow Cooker Orange Chicken — 113
Smothered Mexican Chicken — 114
Hamburger Stir Fry — 115
Sheet Pan Chicken or Fish — 116
Bacon Cheeseburger Casserole — 117
DLG Boneless Wings — 118
Burrito Bowl — 119
Peanut Thai Chicken Stir Fry — 120
Zucchini Noodle Spaghetti — 122
Meatloaf — 123
Sweet Potato Noodle Stir Fry — 124
Chicken Fajitas With Cilantro Lime Sauce — 126
DLG Chicken Fingers — 128
Shepherd's Pie — 129
Curry — 130
Almond Flour Crust Pizza — 131
Vegetable Lasagna — 132
Stuffed Peppers — 133
Slow Cooker Beef + Broccoli — 134
Brisket Tacos — 135
Lemon Garlic Fish — 136
Stuffed Sweet Potatoes — 137
Zucchini Burrito Boats — 138
Almond Crusted Fish — 139
Teriyaki Sheet Pan Chicken + Veggies — 140

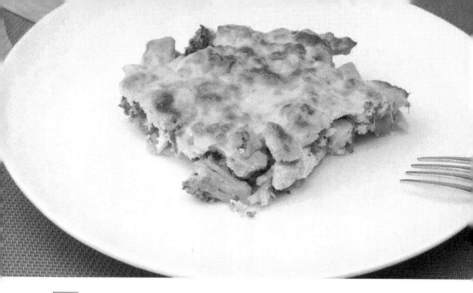

DLG Casserole

Serves 6 | 60 Minutes

4 organic chicken breasts

2 bunches of broccoli

8 oz shredded organic cheddar cheese

1 bunch green onion (sliced)

Salt, pepper, garlic powder (to taste)

2 tbsp natural multipurpose seasoning

1/2 cup Vegenaise (or mayo with no bad oil)

1 1/2 cups sliced almonds

1/2 stick butter

Boil chicken until cooked through. Season and cut into cubes. Steam broccoli until tender. Combine all ingredients except almonds and butter and mix well. Press into a 9 13 baking dish. Sprinkle with almonds on top and drizzle with melted butter. Bake at 375 degrees F for approximately 30 minutes.

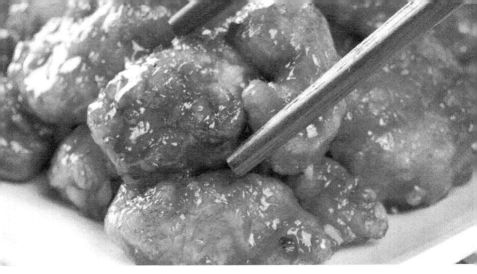

Slow Cooker Orange Chicken

Serves 4 | 10 Minutes + Up To 4 Hours In Slow Cooker

Put the chicken pieces in the bottom of the slow cooker. In a bowl, whisk all of the other ingredients (except sesame seeds) well to remove clumps. Pour the mixture over the chicken and toss to coat. Then cook on low for 3-4 hours, or cook on high for 1 1/2-2 hours. If the sauce seems too thick, add additional orange juice to loosen it up. Top with sesame seeds. In our house, we serve this over cauliflower rice!

Anti-Inflammatory Plan Tip: Coconut sugar and arrowroot (cassava flour) are options for this plan, in moderation, if no known sensitivities. Also, remove crushed red pepper on this plan.

2 lbs organic chicken breasts (cut into bite-sized pieces)

1 cup orange juice (freshly squeezed)

2 tsp zest from the orange

1/2 cup Braggs liquid aminos or coconut aminos

1/4 cup coconut sugar

3 tbsp arrowroot powder

2 tbsp rice vinegar

1 tbsp fresh ginger (grated - or ginger root powder)

2 cloves garlic (minced - or garlic powder)

1 tbsp sesame oil

1/2 tsp crushed red pepper (optional)

2 tbsp sesame seeds

Cauliflower rice (for serving, optional)

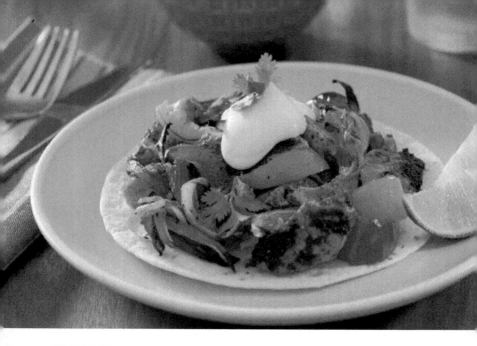

Smothered Mexican Chicken

Serves 6 | 60 Minutes

2 organic chicken breasts

Salt, pepper, cumin, garlic powder, and chili powder (to taste)

3 tbsp coconut oil

1 green bell pepper (sliced)

1 red bell pepper (sliced)

1 red onion (sliced)

1 can black beans

1 cup organic cheddar cheese (shredded)

2 tbsp salsa (watch ingredients)

Optional toppings: sour cream, cilantro, avocado

Tortilla shells (optional - for serving)

Season chicken with spices. Bake the chicken at 350 degrees F in small baking dish until cooked through, approximately 45 minutes. Sauté veggies in coconut oil in a frying pan. Place the sautéed veggies on top of the chicken once done. Cover with black beans. Top with cheese. Place back in the oven to melt the cheese. Top with optional toppings and salsa.

Low Carb Plan Tip:
My family likes to smother a whole chicken breast with the ingredients and skip the tortillas. You may chop up the chicken and serve with either spelt tortillas or another good brand like Siete tortillas.

Vegetarian Plan Tip:
Remove the chicken breasts and add more vegetables.

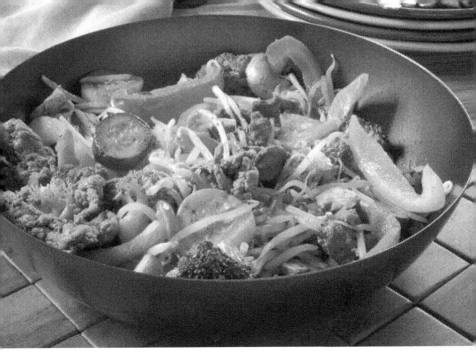

Hamburger Stir Fry

Serves 2 | 30 Minutes

Brown hamburger in coconut oil until cooked. Add vegetables and seasonings and sauté until tender. Can serve over cauliflower rice, rice noodles or cooked bean noodles, if preferred.

Anti-Inflammatory Plan Tip:
Avoid peppers and replace coconut oil with avocado oil, if sensitive.

Low Carb Plan Tip:
Avoid rice noodles and serve with either the cauliflower rice or bean noodles.

Vegetarian Plan Tip:
Yes, you can have hamburger stir fry, just remove the hamburger and add more vegetables.

3 tbsp coconut oil

1 lb grass-fed beef

Salt, pepper, garlic powder (to taste)

3 tbsp Braggs liquid aminos (more or less to taste)

Variety of vegetables: broccoli, bell peppers, onion, snap peas, zucchini, squash, mushrooms, peas, cauliflower carrots, etc. - or whatever vegetables you have on hand

Cauliflower rice, rice noodles or bean noodles (for serving)

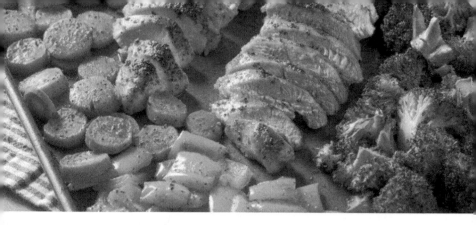

Sheet Pan Chicken or Fish + Veggies

Serves 2 | 40 Minutes

2 organic chicken breasts or thighs (or try a fresh, wild-caught fish)

4-6 tbsp avocado oil or olive oil

Combo of spices to the right

6 rainbow carrots (sliced in half)

1 bunch asparagus (cut into bite-sized pieces)

1 zucchini (cut into thick chunks)

1 yellow squash (cut into thick chunks)

1/2 lb brussels sprouts (cut bottom off and slice in half)

1 red onion (diced)

3 garlic cloves (crushed - optional)

In a large bowl combine all chopped veggies and chicken/fish. Pour oil and spices* over veggie and chicken mixture and coat evenly. Place on a lined baking sheet and bake at 400 degrees F for approximately 30 minutes until chicken is fully cooked through and veggies are soft.

Feel free to use whatever veggies you have on hand and need to use up.

*You can use any combo of the following spices you have on hand:
1 tsp cumin
1 tsp garlic powder
1 tsp onion granules
1 1/2 tsp paprika
2 tsp fresh thyme
2 tsp fresh rosemary
1/4 tsp ground ginger
Salt and pepper, to taste

Low Carb Plan Tip:
Use less or no carrots and more of the other veggies.

Vegetarian Plan Tip:
Remove chicken, roast more veggies, and serve with cauliflower rice or quinoa.

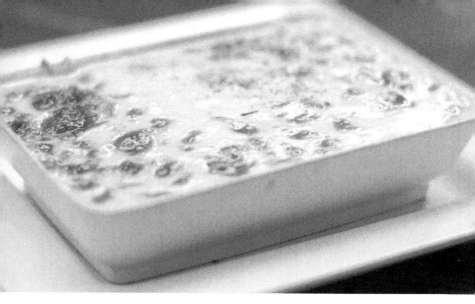

Bacon Cheeseburger Casserole

Serves 6 | 60 Minutes

Make cauliflower mashed tatoes and set aside. Cook turkey bacon in large skillet and set aside. Keep the bacon grease in pan. Add ground beef / turkey to the same skillet and cook until browned. Add the seasonings and set aside. For the sauce: add butter to the same pan and stir in the flour over low heat. Cook until the flour has absorbed the butter and then add heavy cream and mustard. Cook until the sauce thickens.

In a 9x13 baking dish, place half of the sauce on the bottom. Next, spread the cauliflower tatoes as evenly as possible. Sprinkle half of the bag of cheese over the tatoes. Sprinkle on the ground beef. Pour the other half of the sauce over the beef. Sprinkle remaining cheddar cheese over the sauce and sprinkle the top with the bacon. Cover and bake at 350 degrees F for approximately 30 minutes. Allow to cool a bit before serving.

1 head cauliflower (cooked per Mashed Cauliflower Tatoes recipe on page 145)

1 package of turkey bacon (cooked and cut into bite-sized pieces)

1 1/2 lb grass-fed beef (or organic ground turkey)

Salt, pepper, garlic powder, onion powder (optional)

Sauce:
2 tbsp butter

1/3 cup coconut flour

1 1/2 cup organic heavy cream

3 tbsp yellow mustard

1 8 oz package organic cheddar cheese

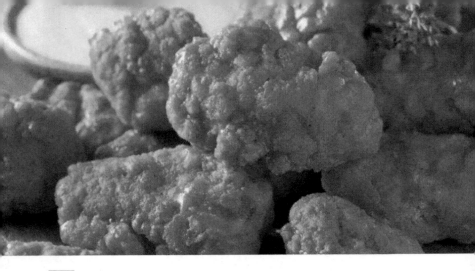

DLG Boneless Wings
Serves 4 | 60 Minutes

1-2 cups coconut oil (for frying)

1 cup of almond or coconut flour

2 tsp sea salt

1/2 tsp of pepper

1/2 tsp cayenne pepper

1/4 tsp garlic powder

1/2 tsp paprika

2 organic eggs

1 cup of almond milk, coconut milk or organic half and half (Match with flour used)

3 organic chicken breasts

1/4 cup of hot sauce or low carb barbecue sauce

3 tbsp of butter

Heat oil in a deep-fryer or large saucepan to 375 degrees F. Combine flour, salt, pepper, cayenne pepper, garlic powder, and paprika in a large bowl. Whisk together the egg and milk in a small bowl. Dip each piece of chicken in the egg mixture, and then roll in the flour blend. Refrigerate or freeze breaded chicken for 20 minutes.

Fry chicken in the hot oil, in batches. Cook until the exterior is nicely browned, and the juices run clear, 5 to 6 minutes a batch.

Combine hot sauce and butter in a small saucepan. Melt the butter into the sauce on low heat and stir. Put cooked chicken into the covered bowl and pour over the hot sauce mix or BBQ and shake gently to coat.

We serve ours with the Homemade Ranch Recipe (page 165).

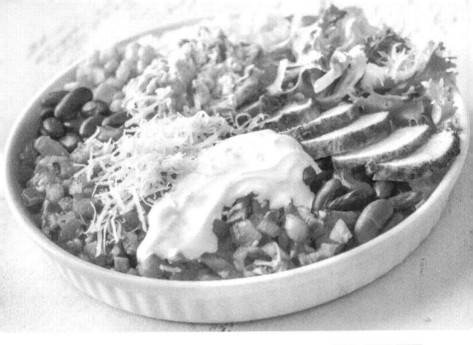

Burrito Bowl

Serves 2 | 20 Minutes

In a pan melt coconut oil or butter. Cook chicken on medium/low heat in the oil until cooked through. Add black beans, corn, and all seasonings. Simmer 2-3 more minutes. Dish up into bowl and top with the toppings.

Anti-Inflammatory Plan Tip:
Coconut oil, beans and corn are options for this plan, in moderation, if no known sensitivities. Avoid chili powder, butter, cheese, and sour cream.

Vegetarian Plan Tip:
Remove chicken and add more good fats such as guacamole.

2 tbsp coconut oil or butter

2 organic chicken breasts (cut into chunks)

1 15 oz can of black beans

1 15 oz can of organic non-GMO corn

3 tsp cumin

2 tsp chili powder

Salt, pepper, garlic salt (to taste)

Optional toppings: organic shredded cheddar cheese, organic sour cream, cilantro, avocado, shredded lettuce, and guacamole (see recipe page 201)

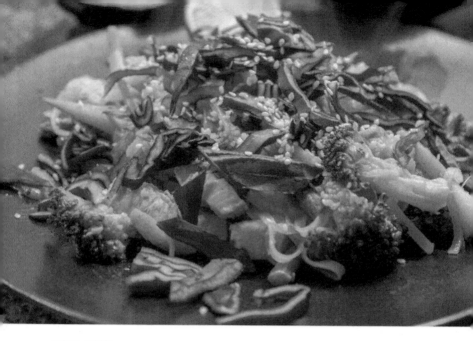

Peanut Thai Chicken Stir Fry
Serves 2-4 | 40 Minutes

2 tbsp coconut oil or butter

2 organic chicken breasts

1 cup broccoli (cut into chunks)

1 cup purple cabbage (shredded)

1/2 cup red bell pepper (sliced)

1/2 cup carrots (shredded)

1/2 cup red onion (sliced)

Sea salt, pepper, garlic powder (to taste)

Cauliflower rice or quinoa (for serving)

1/2 cup cilantro

(Continued on next page)

In a pan melt 2 tbsp coconut oil or butter. Cut chicken into chunks and cook on medium/low heat in the oil until cooked through. Add the vegetables and about 1 tbsp water to help cook the vegetables. Cook until tender. In a saucepan combine the sauce ingredients. On low heat, slowly melt and stir the ingredients until smooth. Add the sauce to the chicken and vegetables and let simmer for a few minutes. Serve over cauliflower rice or quinoa and top with cilantro.

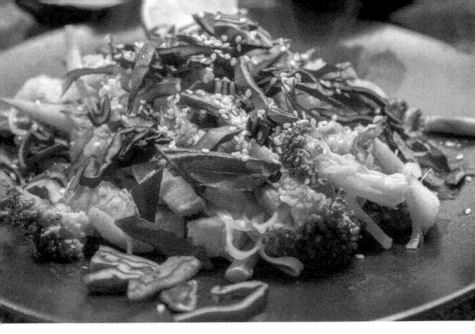

Peanut Thai Chicken Stir Fry

Continued From Previous Page

In a saucepan combine the sauce ingredients. On low heat, slowly melt and stir the ingredients until smooth.

Low Carb Plan Tip:
Avoid serving over quinoa and go for the cauliflower rice.

Vegetarian Plan Tip:
Approved for vegetarians that eat eggs and/or dairy. Remove the chicken and serve over quinoa.

Sauce:
1 cup almond butter or organic valencia peanut butter

4 tbsp butter

1/8 cup chili oil

1/2 cup water

1/4 cup tamari

1/2 juice of a lime

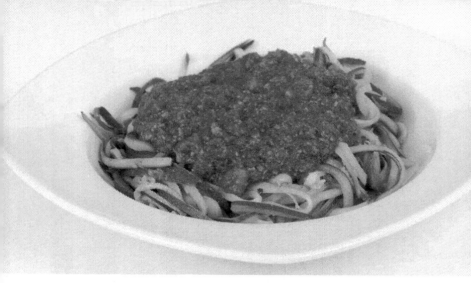

Zucchini Noodle Spaghetti
Serves 2 | 25 Minutes

1 lb grass-fed beef

1 zucchini (cut into long thin strands, use a spiralizer, or buy pre-spiralized noodles)

1 jar spaghetti sauce (or make your own below)

Spaghetti Sauce:
1 can organic tomato sauce

1 can organic diced tomatoes

1-6 oz can organic tomato paste

1 tsp dried basil

1/2 tsp dried oregano

1/2 tsp garlic powder

1/2 tsp onion powder

1/4 tsp ground thyme

Salt and pepper (to taste)

In a large pan, brown hamburger and season with salt and pepper. Once the hamburger is cooked through, add the sauce into the pan. If making your own sauce, you can just put all sauce ingredients right into the pan with hamburger, stir and warm. Mix the zucchini noodles into the sauce mix. If you are spiralizing your own noodles, simply follow the tool's instructions. You may need to press the noodles down a bit to submerge the sauce. Simmer for approximately 10 minutes or until the noodles are tender.

Vegetarian Plan Tip:
Remove ground beef.

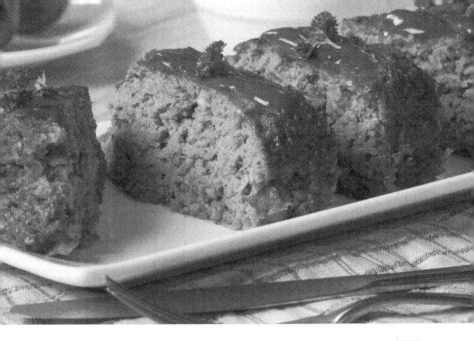

Meatloaf

Serves 4 | 1 1/2 Hours

Mix all ingredients well in a bowl. Transfer to a lightly coconut oil greased loaf pan, pack lightly. Bake 1 hour or until cooked through at 350 degrees F. Can top with a little ketchup, if desired. We like to serve with Mashed Cauliflower Tatoes (see recipe page 145).

Low Carb Plan Tip:
Avoid the healthy crackers and make sure to watch the ingredients in the sauces.

1 1/2 lbs grass-fed beef

1 organic egg

1 small onion (diced)

1/2 cup ketchup or tomato paste (no sugar)

2 tbsp Braggs liquid aminos

2 tsp worcestershire sauce

Salt, pepper, garlic powder (to taste)

Healthy cracker (finely crushed, optional - clean brands such as Simple Mills, Mary's Gone Crackers or Akmak crackers)

Coconut oil (for greasing)

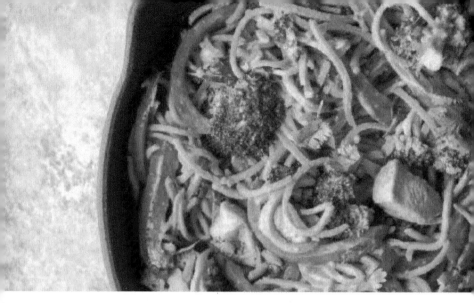

Sweet Potato Noodle Stir Fry Thai or Teriyaki

Serves 2 | 25 Minutes

2 tbsp coconut oil

1 cup pea pods

1 cup yellow onion (sliced)

1 cup broccoli (cut into bite-sized pieces)

1 cup red bell pepper (sliced)

1 can water chestnuts (drained)

1 container of sweet potato or zucchini noodles (pre-made package or use a spiralizing tool and 2 medium sized sweet potatoes/ zucchini)

Cilantro (optional)

2 organic chicken breasts (pre-cooked - optional)

(Continue on next page)

In a large pan sauté all vegetables and chestnuts, except the noodles, in the coconut oil until tender. If using thai sauce, add to a saucepan, combining all ingredients and warming on low heat. Stir until a smooth consistency. Once the vegetables are tender add your sweet potato noodles and pour the sauce in the pan. Simmer for approximately 10 minutes on medium/low to medium heat until the noodles are tender. Top with cilantro or add chicken to this dish to complete it!

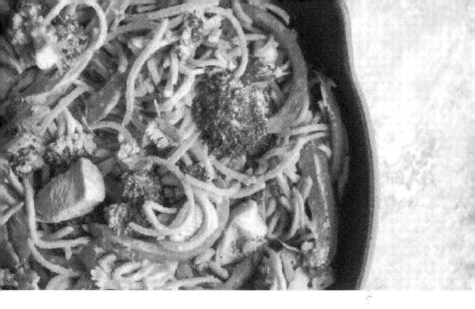

Sweet Potato Noodle Stir Fry
Thai or Teriyaki

Continued From Previous Page

Thai Sauce:
Combine in bowl and whisk together.

Anti-Inflammatory Plan Tip:
Coconut, almond, cashew, and flax milk or butter are options for this plan, in moderation, if no known sensitivities. Avoid bell pepper and sriracha/chili oil all together.

Low Carb Plan Tip:
Instead of sweet potato noodles, use zucchini noodles.

Vegetarian Plan Tip:
Remove chicken and add more veggies.

Thai Sauce:
1/4 cup raw almond butter or organic Valencia peanut butter

2 tbsp Braggs liquid aminos (or similar soy sauce alternative)

1/2 tsp ground ginger

1/2 tsp garlic powder

1 tbsp sriracha sauce or chili oil

1 tsp sesame oil

1/2-3/4 cup coconut milk from the carton (or light coconut milk from can)

Teriyaki Sauce:
I buy Coconut Secret brand teriyaki sauce

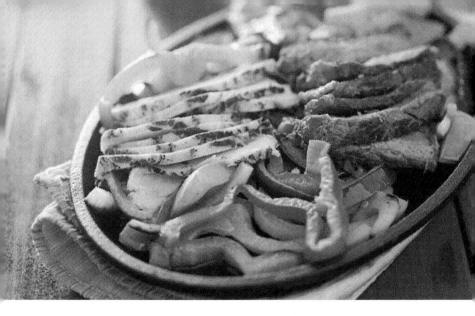

Fajitas With Cilantro-Lime Sauce

Serves 2 | 30 Minutes

Fajita Seasoning:
3 tbsp chili powder

2 tsp onion powder

2 tsp garlic powder

2 tbsp ground cumin

2 tsp sea salt

1 1/2 tbsp smoked paprika
(optional)

1/2 tsp cayenne pepper
(optional)

Cilantro-Lime Sauce:
1 cup plain, grass-fed yogurt
or full-fat greek yogurt

1 tbsp homemade fajita
seasoning

1 clove garlic (finely minced -
or 1/2 tsp garlic powder)

2 tbsp fresh cilantro (finely
chopped)

2 tbsp fresh lime juice

Salt and pepper (to taste)

Prepare the fajita seasoning by combining all ingredients in a small bowl and stirring until thoroughly blended. Save any excess in an airtight container for later use if desired or use extra in the recipe.

Prepare the cilantro-lime sauce by thoroughly combining all ingredients in a small bowl. Cover and place in the refrigerator until ready to use.

Anti-Inflammatory Plan Tip: You may sacrifice some taste but remove chili powder, cayenne pepper, and paprika from the fajita seasoning. Avoid cilantro-lime sauce and peppers, as well. Replace coconut oil with avocado oil, if sensitive.

Vegetarian Plan Tip: Remove meat and add extra veggies and healthy fats like guacamole.

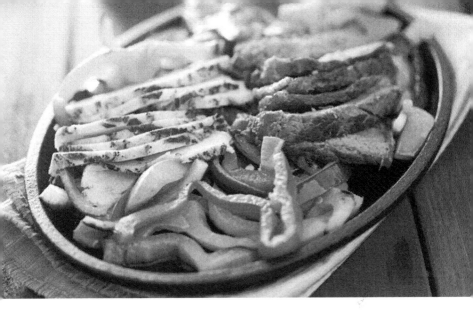

Fajitas With Cilantro-Lime Sauce

Continued From Previous Page

Heat the coconut oil in a large pan over medium/low heat. Cook the chicken until cooked through. Add the bell peppers and onion to the pan and season with salt and pepper, to taste. Cook for 10-12 minutes or until the onions and peppers are tender. Add the seasoning, and chicken stock to the pan and stir to combine. Cook until heated through and excess liquid is gone, approximately 3-4 minutes. Season with additional salt or fajita seasoning, if desired.

Remove pan from heat and stir in the cilantro and fresh lime juice. To serve, spoon mixture into individual romaine lettuce leaves and top with a drizzle of cilantro-lime sauce.

Fajitas:
2 tbsp coconut oil

2 organic chicken breasts (cut into stripes) - can substitute for steak or wild-caught fish

1 red, green, yellow and orange bell pepper (sliced thin)

1/2 small red onion (sliced thin)

Salt and pepper (to taste)

3 tbsp homemade fajita seasoning (on previous page)

1/4 cup organic chicken bone broth (optional – can use water too)

1/4 cup fresh cilantro (chopped)

2 tbsp fresh lime juice (optional)

Romaine lettuce or Siete brand shells (for serving)

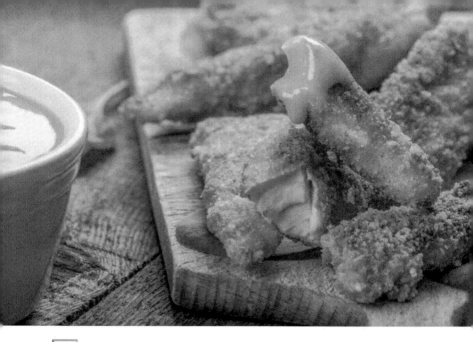

DLG Chicken Fingers

Serves 2 | 20 Minutes

1 cup almond or coconut flour

Salt, pepper, garlic powder (to taste)

2 organic chicken breasts (cut into strips)

2 organic eggs (beaten)

6 tbsp coconut oil

Homemade ranch dressing (see recipe page 165)

In a small bowl mix flour and seasoning, set aside. Dip chicken strips into egg and then the flour mixture. Be sure they are well coated. Cover the bottom of a frying pan with melted coconut oil. Be sure pan is covered. Fry on medium/low to medium heat until golden brown on both sides and chicken is cooked through.

We love to dip these in the homemade ranch dressing (page 165), a clean ketchup or honey mustard (check ingredients for no added sugar).

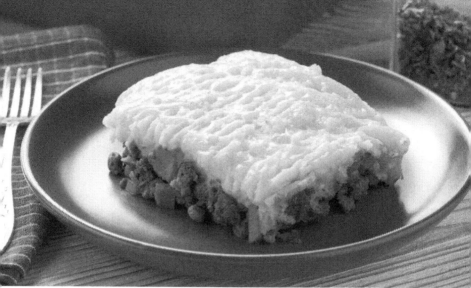

Shepherd's Pie

Ai **LC**

Serves 4 | 60 Minutes

Follow recipe for mashed cauliflower tatoes and set aside.

Brown hamburger, add in onion, carrots, peas and let steam until tender, approximately 10 minutes.

In separate saucepan, simmer beef broth, onion and cauliflower rice for approximately 10 minutes. Remove from heat and add seasonings, worcestershire sauce, and butter. Put all ingredients into a blender and mix until smooth, adding in the arrowroot powder until it becomes a puree.

Pour over the meat and vegetables in an 8x8 baking dish and top with mashed cauliflower tatoes. Cook at 350 degrees F until warm throughout or until top starts to brown.

Anti-Inflammatory Plan Tip:
Sub the butter in the sauce with avocado oil. Arrowroot (cassava) is an option for this plan, in moderation, if no known sensitivities.

Topping:
Mashed Cauliflower Tatoes
(see recipe page 145)

Inside:
1 lb grass-fed beef

1/2 onion (diced)

3 carrots (diced)

1 cup peas

Sauce:
2 cups beef bone broth

1/2 onion (diced)

1 cup cauliflower rice

Salt, pepper, and garlic powder (to taste)

2 tsp worcestershire sauce

4 tbsp butter

1/2 cup arrowroot powder

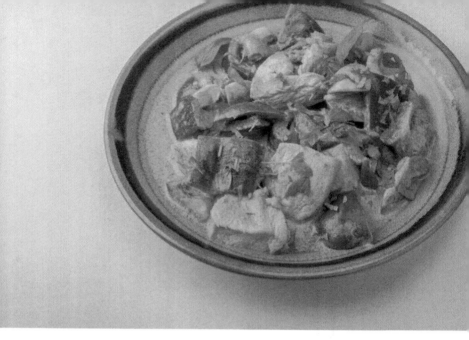

Curry

Serves 2 | 45 Minutes

2 organic chicken breasts

1 can coconut milk

2 cups broccoli

1 red or green bell pepper (cubed)

1 cup mushrooms

1 onion (diced)

3 tbsp curry powder

1 tsp garlic (minced - or garlic powder)

1 tsp ginger (minced - can also use powder)

Salt and pepper (to taste)

Cauliflower rice (for serving - optional)

In a large frying pan cut chicken into cubes and cook until almost cooked all the way through, approximately 10-15 minutes. Add coconut milk, vegetables, and all seasonings. Simmer 15-20 minutes until vegetables are tender. Can enjoy over cauliflower rice if desired.

Anti-Inflammatory Plan Tip: Avoid bell peppers. Coconut milk is an option for this plan, in moderation, if no known sensitivities.

Vegetarian Plan Tip: Remove chicken and add more veggies like broccoli.

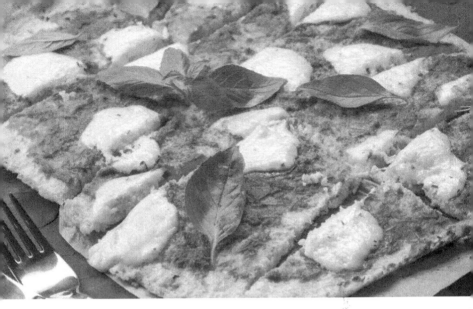

Almond Flour Crust Pizza

Serves 2 | 45 Minutes

Mix all crust ingredients together until it forms a ball. Roll the dough into a 1/4 inch pizza crust on a sheet pan lined with parchment paper. Can use oil or butter on hands to make dough less sticky. Bake at 350 degrees F for 10-15 minutes. Top with your favorite healthy pizza ingredients, cheese, and return to the oven for another 10-15 minutes or until cheese is melted.

Vegetarian Plan Tip:
Approved for vegetarians that eat eggs and/or dairy.

1 1/4 cups almond flour

1/4 cup ground flax meal

1/2 tsp sea salt

1/4 tsp baking soda

1 egg (beaten)

1 tbsp olive oil

1 package organic mozzarella cheese

Your favorite, optional pizza toppings: pizza sauce, bell peppers, onion, mushrooms, olives, hamburger, turkey bacon, etc.

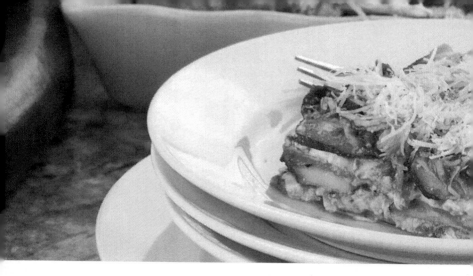

Vegetable Lasagna

Serves 6 | 90 Minutes

1 large eggplant (sliced into 1/4 inch rounds)

1/2 lb mushrooms (sliced)

3 zucchini (sliced length-wise into 1/4 inch slices)

2 red bell peppers (cut into 6 pieces each)

3 tbsp olive oil

1 clove garlic (minced)

Salt and pepper (to taste)

1-15 oz container of ricotta cheese (optional)

1/4 cup parmesan cheese (grated)

1 organic egg

1 jar pasta sauce

2 cups organic shredded mozzarella cheese

3 tsp basil

Spread eggplant and mushrooms onto a baking pan. Place zucchini and red peppers on a second pan. Brush oil and garlic over both sides of the vegetables and sprinkle with salt and pepper. Bake at 400 degrees F for 20-30 minutes, turning half way through until vegetables are tender and pepper edges are browned. In a bowl, combine ricotta cheese, parmesan cheese, and egg. Spread about 1/2 cup pasta sauce in a 9 13 baking dish. Layer with half the ricotta cheese mixture, half of the vegetables, a third of the pasta sauce and 2/3 cup of the mozzarella cheese. Sprinkle with basil and repeat the layers. Top with remaining pasta sauce. Cover and bake at 350 degrees F for 30-40 minutes. Uncover and sprinkle with remaining cheese. Bake 5-10 minutes until cheese is melted. Let stand for 10 minutes before cutting.

Vegetarian Plan Tip: Approved for vegetarians that eat eggs and/or dairy.

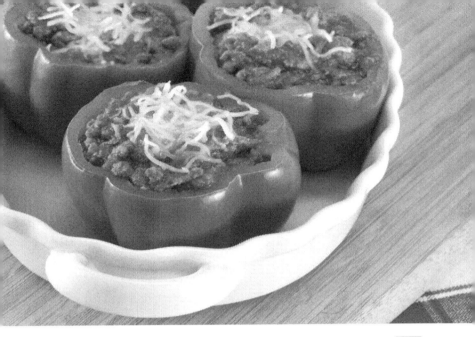

Stuffed Peppers

Serves 4 | 60 Minutes

Preheat oven to 400 degrees F. Sauté meat and onions over medium/low heat in pan until browned. Meanwhile, place peppers cut side down on baking sheet and bake until tender, approximately 20-25 minutes. Add seasoning, aminos, and diced tomatos to the pan with meat and onions and stir together. Fill pepper halves with the beef mixture. Bake 5-10 minutes or until heated through. Can top with parmesan or any cheese, if desired. Can serve with Mashed Cauliflower Tatoes (page 145) or quinoa.

Low Carb Plan Tip:
Avoid quinoa and stick with Mashed Cauliflower Tatoes.

1 1/2 lbs grass-fed beef

1 onion (diced)

4 red, green, yellow, or orange bell peppers (top cut off)

Salt, pepper, garlic powder (to taste)

2 tbsp Braggs liquid aminos

1 small can organic italian-style diced tomatoes

Organic parmesan cheese or cheese of choice (optional)

Mashed Cauliflower Tatoes (see recipe on page 145 or 1/2 cup of cooked quinoa - for serving - optional)

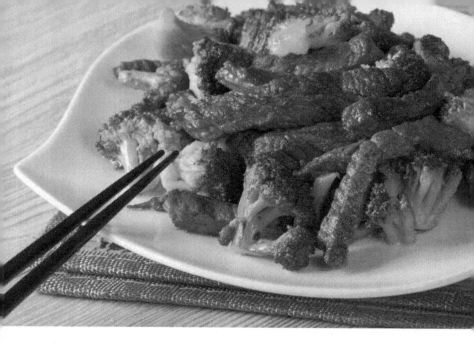

Slow Cooker Beef and Broccoli

Serves 2 | 6-8 Hours In Slow Cooker

1 lb grass-fed steak (ribeye works well)

1/4-1/2 cup coconut aminos

2 tbsp apple cider vinegar

2 tsp coconut oil

1 head of broccoli

1 tbsp sesame seeds

Salt, pepper, garlic powder (to taste)

1/2 tsp red pepper flakes (optional)

Cook on low for approximately 6-8 hours with all Ingredients mixed together (except the broccoli and sesame seeds). Add the broccoli approximately an hour before eating and cook until tender. Serve with sesame seeds on top.

Anti-Inflammatory Plan Tip: Replace coconut oil with avocado oil, if sensitive. Avoid red pepper flakes.

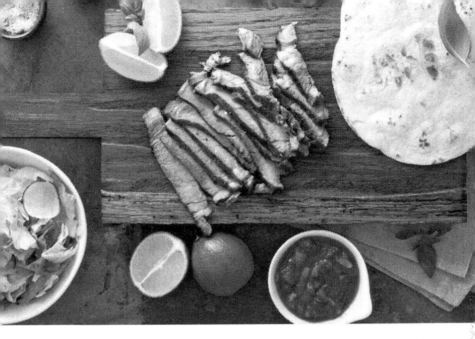

Brisket Tacos

Serves 4 | 6-8 In Slow Cooker

Put brisket meat in a slow cooker on medium for 6-8 hours with a very small amount of water and approximately 1/3 of the jar of salsa verde (cook until tender and easy to pull apart with a fork). Once meat is done put in shells, wrap or on bed of spinach and top with cheese and salsa and any other desired toppings!

Anti-Inflammatory Plan Tip:
Avoid cheese, dairy, and tortilla options.

Low Carb Plan Tip:
You can put on a bed of spinach or in cabbage cups instead of making tacos

2 lbs grass-fed brisket (approximately 1/4-1/2 pound per person)

1 jar salsa verde

Cotija cheese (shredded)

Optional toppings: avocado, sour cream, red onion, cilantro, lime, shredded lettuce

Optional wraps: Siete brand wraps, organic whole grain spelt tortillas, coconut wraps, Ezekiel brand tortillas or opt for serving over a bed of spinach

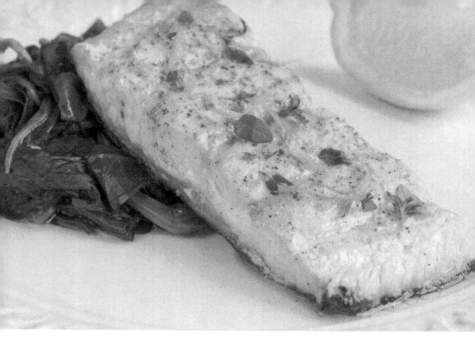

Lemon Garlic Fish
Serves 2 | 20 Minutes

3 tbsp butter

1 tbsp garlic (minced - or 1 tsp garlic powder)

2 pieces of wild-caught fish of choice (salmon works well)

1 lemon (zest and juice)

1 tbsp ground cumin

Sea salt and pepper (to taste)

Optional: parsley (for topping)

Cauliflower rice, quinoa, or bean noodle pasta (for serving)

Melt butter in a large frying pan over medium heat. Add garlic and sauté for 1-2 minutes, stirring. Add fish, lemon zest, lemon juice, and cumin to the pan and cook for approximately 5 minutes on each side or until cooked through. Can also "flash fry" to crisp the outside of the fish in a small frying pan of olive oil on medium heat after it is cooked through in other pan. Serve over cauliflower rice, on a bed of quinoa, or over your favorite bean noodle pasta. Drizzle some of the pan juice over each piece of fish and garnish with fresh parsley, if desired.

Anti-Inflammatory Plan Tip: Sub the butter for avocado oil.

Low Carb Plan Tip: Stick with serving over cauliflower rice.

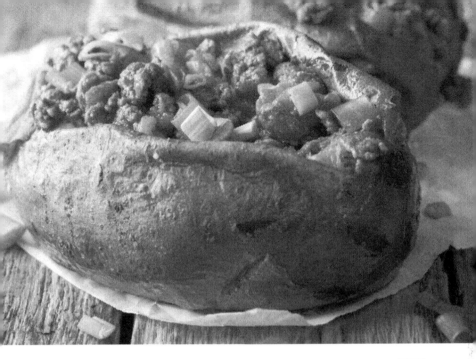

Stuffed Sweet Potatoes

Serves 2 | 60 Minutes

Prick the sweet potatoes with a fork all over. Bake at 425 degree F for approximately 40 minutes or until soft enough to cut open.

While the potatoes are baking, brown the hamburger with the seasonings and add the tomatoes at the end to warm. Once the potatoes are done and "cool" enough, cut open lengthwise, pull it apart wide enough to "stuff" it with the meat mixture, top with cheese, and bake for approximately 5 more minutes or until the cheese is melted.

Anti-Inflammatory Plan Tip:
Sweet potatoes and tomatoes are options for this plan, in moderation, if no known sensitivities. Avoid chili powder and cheese all together.

2 medium sweet potatoes

1/2-3/4 lb grass-fed beef

2 tsp ground cumin

1 tsp garlic powder

1 tsp chili powder

Sea salt and pepper (to taste)

1 cup canned diced tomatoes

1 cup shredded organic pepper jack cheese

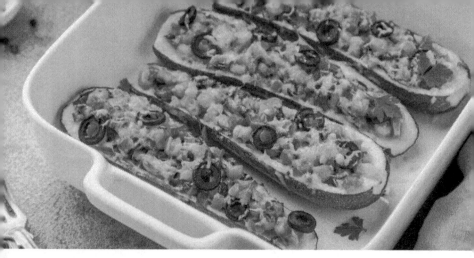

Zucchini Burrito Boats

Serves 2 | 60 Minutes

2 large zucchini

1 tbsp olive oil

1/2 lb grass-fed beef

1/4 red onion (diced)

1/2 cup red bell pepper (diced)

1 jalapeño (cored and diced)

1/2 can black beans (drained)

1/2 cup organic non-GMO corn (optional)

1/2 cup salsa

2 tsp cumin

1 tsp chili powder

Sea salt, pepper, garlic powder (to taste)

1 cup shredded organic monterey or pepper jack cheese

Optional toppings: organic sour cream, cilantro, and black olives

Slice the zucchini in half, lengthwise. Using a melon baller or a spoon, scoop out the center of each zucchini. Brush both sides with a little olive oil and place them skin side down in a casserole dish.

In a large frying pan, brown the beef in a little olive oil until mostly cooked. Add the onion and peppers and cook an additional 5 minutes or until the vegetables are tender. Add the beans, corn, salsa, and the seasonings and cook another approximately 5 minutes. Spoon the meat filling into each zucchini. Cover with foil and bake for approximately 20-25 minutes at 400 degrees F. Remove the foil and top with cheese and cook for another 5 minutes or until the cheese is melted. Top with cilantro and organic sour cream and enjoy.

Anti-Inflammatory Plan Tip: Avoid peppers, chili powder, cheese and sour cream. Black beans are an option for this plan, in moderation, if no known senstivies.

Vegetarian Plan Tip: Just remove the beef and enjoy!

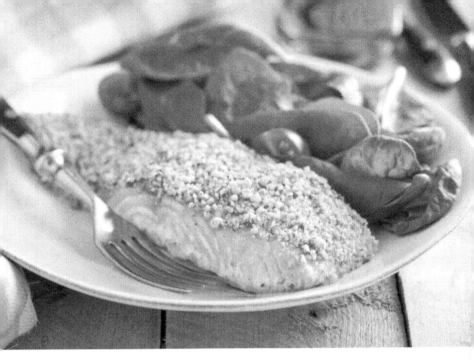

Almond Crusted Fish

Serves 2 | 20 Minutes

Mix almond, parmesan cheese, salt and pepper in a small bowl. Combine melted butter and garlic powder in another small bowl. Brush the butter mixture on both sides of the fish and place on a butter greased baking dish or sheet, bottom side up. Broil for approximately 4-5 minutes. Flip the fish over and sprinkle with the nut and cheese mixture. Broil for approximately 3-5 more minutes or until cooked through and topping is golden.

Anti-Inflammatory Plan Tip: Almonds are an option for this plan, in moderation, if no known sensitivities. Avoid the parmesan cheese. Sub the butter for avocado oil.

1/4 cup almonds (finely chopped)

1/4 cup grated parmesan cheese

Sea salt and pepper (to taste)

1/4 cup butter (melted)

1 1/2 tsp garlic powder

2 pieces of wild-caught fish (tilapia works well)

Optional: lemon wedges or fresh parsley (for garnish)

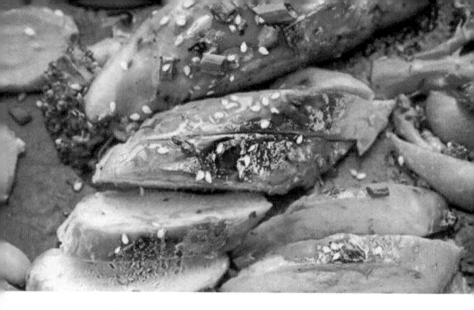

Sheet Pan Teriyaki Chicken + Veggies

Serves 2 | 45 Minutes

2 organic chicken breasts or thighs (or a wild-caught fish)

2 cups broccoli florets

1/2 lb carrots (sliced into thick slices)

1 cup snap peas

4 tbsp Coconut Secret brand aminos (teriyaki flavored)

2 tbsp olive oil

1 tbsp sesame oil (optional, can use all olive oil)

2 tsp sriracha sauce (optional - or hot sauce)

2 cloves garlic (minced - or 1/2 tsp garlic powder)

Green onions + sesame seeds (optional for topping)

(Continued on next page)

Combine ingredients and make Teriyaki sauce on the next page. Slice the chicken breasts in half, long way to thin them out. Toss chicken and veggies in teriyaki sauce and add to a sheet pan in a single layer. May need to drizzle more oil on the vegetables, if desired. Bake at 375 degrees F for approximately 30 minutes or until chicken is cooked and vegetables are browned. Top with green onion and sesame seeds, if desired.

Anti-Inflammatory Plan Tip: Avoid sriracha/hot sauce.

Low Carb Plan Tip: Remove the sweetener (honey/maple syrup) and try coconut sugar, xylitol, or stevia, to taste.

Vegetarian Plan Tip: Remove chicken and add more veggies.

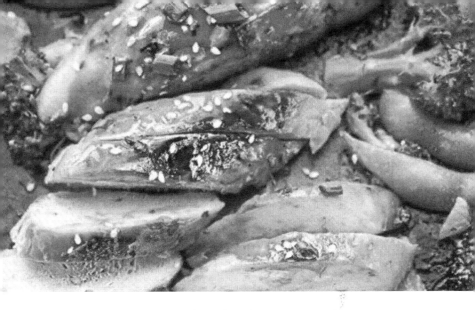

Sheet Pan Teriyaki Chicken + Veggies

Continued From Previous Page

In a saucepan over medium heat, whisk together all ingredients until well combined. Bring to a simmer, stirring frequently, until sauce thickens and bubbles. Remove from heat and toss in chicken and vegetables to coat.

Teriyaki Sauce:
1/2 cup Braggs liquid aminos

3 tbsp local raw honey

3 tbsp rice wine vinegar

1 tbs sesame oil

2 garlic cloves (minced - or 1/2 tsp garlic powder)

3/4 tsp ginger (grated - or ginger root powder)

1 tbsp arrowroot powder

1/4 cup water

Salt and pepper (to taste)

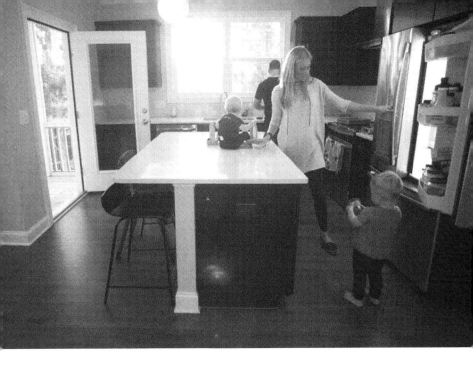

SIDE DISHES

Roasted Broccoli   144

Mashed Cauliflower Tatoes   145

Brussels Sprouts (+ with Balsamic Glaze option)   146

Cauliflower Fried Rice   147

Simple Sautéed Sweet Potatoes   148

Zucchini Fries (Vegetable Fries)   149

Garlic Cheddar Biscuits   150

Spicy Whipped Sweet Potatoes   151

Loaded Mashed Cauliflower   152

Vegetable Medley   153

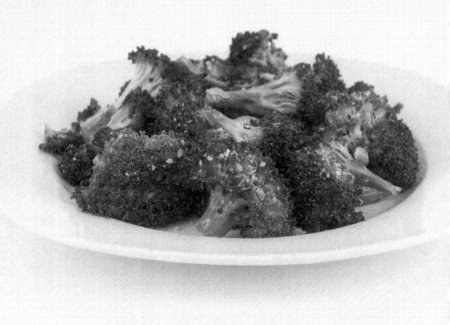

Roasted Broccoli
Serves 2 | 40 Minutes

2 large heads of broccoli

3 tbsp olive oil or avocado oil

Salt and pepper (to taste)

Garlic salt (optional)

Toss the broccoli florets with olive oil and seasoning. Spread them out on a sheet pan and roast at 425 degrees F until the edges are crispy and the stems are tender. Approximately 30 minutes. Can broil them at the end if want them to be more crisp.

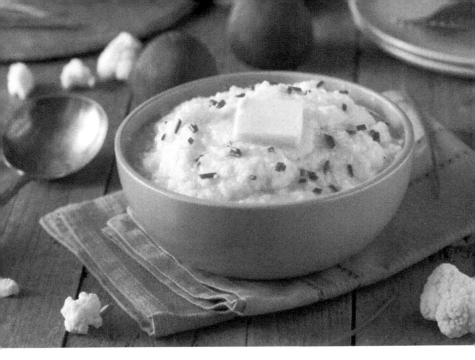

Mashed Cauliflower Tatoes

Serves 2 | 20 Minutes

Steam cauliflower in steamer until tender. Then mix cauliflower, butter and seasonings in a blender until smooth.

Anti-Inflammatory Plan Tip:
Sub the butter for avocado oil.

Vegetarian Plan Tip:
Approved for vegetarians that eat eggs and/or dairy.

1 head cauliflower

4 tbsp butter

Salt and pepper (to taste)

Garlic powder (optional)

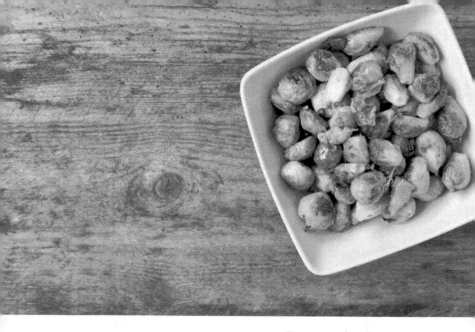

Brussels Sprouts
+ With Balsamic Glaze Option

Serves 2 | 40 Minutes

1 bag of fresh or frozen brussels sprouts (if fresh, cut end off and cut in half)

3 tbsp olive oil

Salt and pepper (to taste)

Garlic powder (to taste)

Organic parmesan cheese (optional)

Balsamic glaze (optional):
1 tbsp balsamic vinegar

1 tbsp local raw honey

Toss the brussels sprouts with olive oil and seasonings. Spread them out and bake at 425 degrees F until tender and outsides are starting to brown. Approximately 30 minutes. Can broil them at the end if you would like them to be more crisp.

Balsamic Glaze Option:
Drizzle balsamic vinegar and honey over the brussels sprouts and stir until coated.

Anti-Inflammatory Plan Tip:
Avoid the cheese.

Low Carb Plan Tip:
Remove the sweetener (honey/maple syrup) and try coconut sugar, xylitol, or stevia, to taste.

Vegetarian Plan Tip:
Avoid cheese, if necessary.

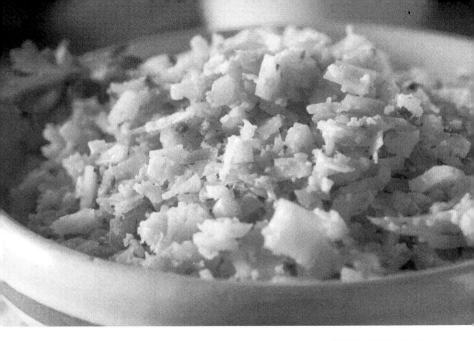

Cauliflower Fried Rice

Serves 2 | 40 Minutes

Sauté veggies (except peas) in butter and garlic on medium heat until tender. If using fresh cauliflower, put in food processor until rice consistency. Add the cauliflower rice to pan and mix together. Clear a small opening in the middle of the pan and add the 3 eggs (can add a little extra butter at this point or some olive oil if you want). Add peas in. Mix well and cook until eggs are cooked. Add liquid aminos to taste. Add baked chicken breast for Chicken Fried Rice.

Anti-Inflammatory Plan Tip:
Remove the eggs but the veggies will still taste good without them!

Vegetarian Plan Tip:
Approved for vegetarians that eat eggs and/or dairy.

4 tbsp butter

Garlic powder or 1 minced clove (to taste)

2 carrots (diced)

4 broccoli pieces (diced)

1 head of cauliflower (riced - or 1 bag of cauliflower rice)

1 onion or 2 green onions (diced)

3 organic eggs

Olive oil (optional)

1/2 cup peas

1/4 cup liquid aminos (Braggs or Coconut Secret Coconut Aminos)

Salt and pepper (to taste)

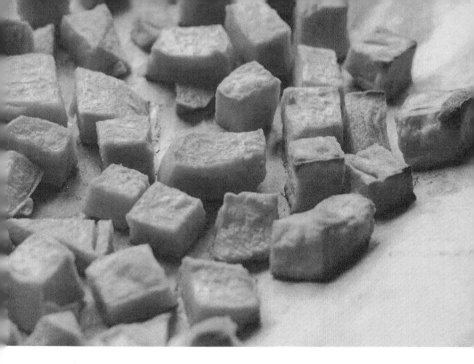

Simple Sautéed Sweet Potatoes

Serves 2 | 20 Minutes

1 large sweet potato (peeled & diced)

3 tbsp coconut oil

Sea salt (to taste)

Cube the sweet potatoes and sauté them in coconut oil on the stove until tender but crispy on the outside. Stirring frequently! Sea salt to top them off and enjoy! That simple!

Anti-Inflammatory Plan Tip: Sweet potatoes and coconut oil are options for this plan, in moderation, if no known sensitivities.

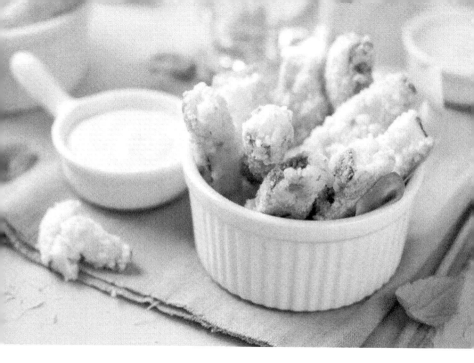

Zucchini Fries (Vegetable Fries)

Serves 1 | 40 Minutes

Combine almond flour and seasoning in a small bowl. Cut zucchini into fry-sized rectangles. Dip zucchini in egg and then dip and cover in flour mixture. Bake on parchment lined baking sheet at 425 degrees F for 20-30 minutes or until brown and crispy.

Vegetarian Plan Tip:
Approved for vegetarians that eat eggs and/or dairy.

1 cup almond flour

Salt, pepper, garlic powder (or cajun spice, check ingredients)

2 organic eggs (beaten)

1 large zucchini (try any vegetable such as asparagus, green beans, etc)

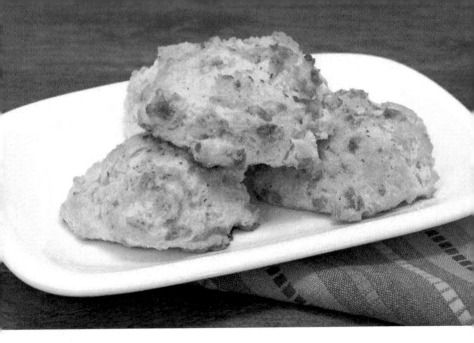

Garlic Cheddar Biscuits
Yields 6 Biscuits | 20 Minutes

2 cups spelt flour (or something similar)

1 tbsp baking powder

1 tsp sea salt

1/3 cup coconut oil (melted)

1 clove of garlic (minced) or 1/2-1 tsp garlic powder

3/4 cup water (hot)

1 tbsp chives (chopped finely)

1/2 cup organic cheddar cheese

2 tbsp butter (if added)

Mix dry ingredients in a bowl. Add garlic, oil and water and mix. Fold in the chives and cheddar cheese. Brush with a little of the left over melted coconut oil or a little butter and sprinkle a little salt on top. Bake 8-10 minutes at 375 degree F.

Anti-Inflammatory Plan Tip: Avoid cheese all together. Coconut oil is an option for this plan, in moderation, if no known sensitivities..

Low Carb Plan Tip: Try subbing ½ almond and ½ coconut flour for the spelt flour.

Vegetarian Plan Tip: Approved for vegetarians that eat eggs and/or dairy.

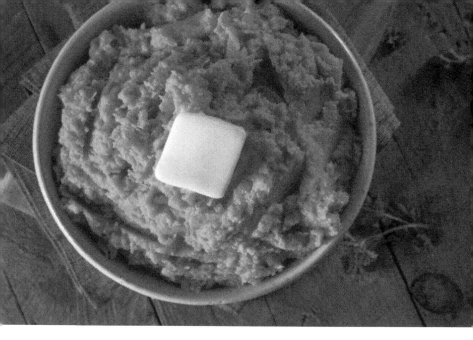

Spicy Whipped Sweet Potatoes

Serves 3-4 | 25 Minutes

Steam or boil peeled and cubed sweet potatoes until softened. Put all ingredients in a high-powered blender and blend until smooth or whip with a hand mixer until smooth. Add more sweet or spicy to your taste!

Vegetarian Plan Tip:
Approved for vegetarians that eat eggs and/or dairy.

2 large sweet potatoes

5 tbsp butter

1/4 tsp cayenne pepper (or to taste)

2 tbsp maple syrup

1/4 tsp cinnamon (optional)

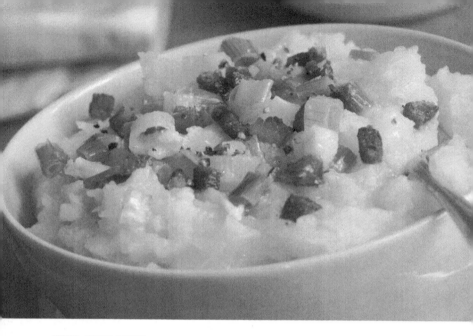

Loaded Mashed Cauliflower

Serves 4 | 30 Minutes

1 head of cauliflower
(chopped into florets)

5 tbsp butter

Salt and pepper (to taste)

4 slices of turkey bacon

1/2 cup organic shredded
cheddar cheese

1 small scallion (sliced thin -
or chives if preferred)

Optional: 2 oz organic cream
cheese and/or 1/4 cup
organic heavy whipping
cream

Steam the cauliflower until the pieces
are tender. Place cauliflower, butter,
salt and pepper, cream cheese, and
whipping cream (if desired) into a
high-powered blender or beat using
a hand mixer. Blend until smooth
consistency.

In a small frying pan, cook the turkey
bacon until brown and done.
Pour the cauliflower into a small
baking dish and top with cheddar
cheese, turkey bacon, and scallions.
Bake at 350 degrees F for
approximately 10-15 minutes or until
the cheese is melted.

Anti-Inflammatory Plan Tip:
Avoid cheese and cream. Sub butter
for avocado oil.

Vegetarian Plan Tip:
Approved for vegetarians that eat
eggs and/or dairy. Remove bacon.

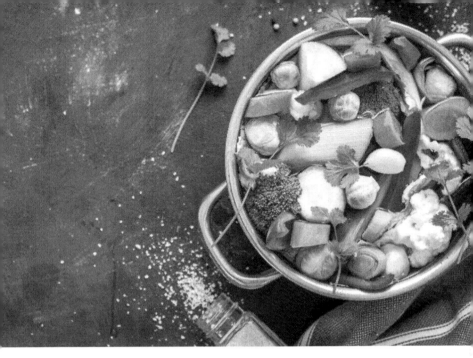

Vegetable Medley

Serves 2 | 20 Minutes

Using medium/low to low heat, sautee vegetables with olive oil and seasonings until tender. Add butter at the end and top with parmesan cheese, if adding.

Of course, feel free to use whatever vegetables you love or have left over and need to use up!

Anti-Inflammatory Plan Tip:
Avoid peppers and cheese all together. Sweet potatos are options for this plan, in moderation, if no known sensitivities.

Low Carb Plan Tip:
Avoid sweet potatoes all together.

Vegetarian Plan Tip:
Approved for vegetarians that eat eggs and/or dairy.

1 cup mini bell peppers (sliced)

8-10 brussels sprouts (ends cut off and halved)

1 small sweet potato (diced)

1/2 cup onion (diced)

1/2 cup organic non-GMO corn (optional)

2 tbsp olive oil

Salt and pepper (to taste)

1 clove of garlic (minced - or garlic powder to taste)

3 tbsp butter (optional)

1/2 cup organic parmesan cheese (grated - optional)

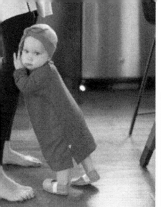
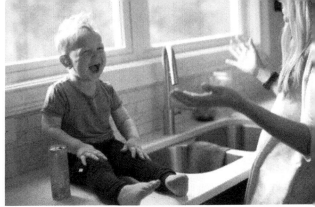

SALADS + SOUPS

Fresh Caprese Salad   156

Simple Chicken Salad   157

Caesar Salad   158

Cobb Salad   159

Mediterranean Quinoa Salad   160

Easy Broccoli Salad   161

Strawberry Goat Cheese Salad   162

Buffalo Chicken Salad   163

BBQ Chicken Salad   164

Homemade Ranch Dressing   165

Chicken Marsala Soup   166

Simple Chili   167

Vegetable + Bean Soup   168

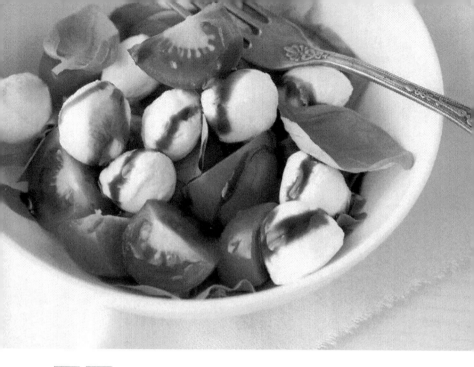

Fresh Caprese Salad

Serves 4 | 15 Minutes

1-10 oz container of grape tomatoes (halved or quarters)

4 oz of fresh mozzarella cheese (cubed)

1/4-1/2 cup fresh basil leaves (sliced)

2 tbsp extra virgin olive oil (to taste)

2 tbsp balsamic vinegar (to taste)

Sea salt (to taste)

In a bowl mix all ingredients together. Sprinkle with sea salt if desired on top. Enjoy!

Vegetarian Plan Tip:
Approved for vegetarians that eat eggs and/or dairy.

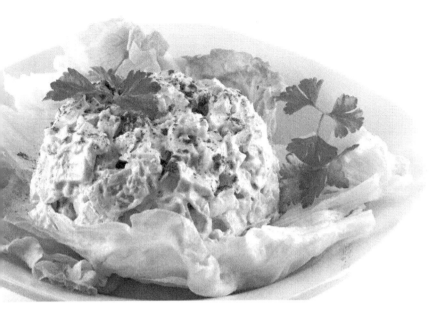

Simple Chicken Salad

Serves 2 | 30 Minutes

Bake or boil chicken until cooked through. Combine all ingredients in a bowl. Serve over a bed of spinach or on romaine lettuce wraps.

Anti-Inflammatory Plan Tip:
Nuts are an option for this plan, in moderation, if no known sensitivities.

Low Carb Plan Tip:
Avoid the optional add-ins.

2 organic chicken breasts (boiled or baked until cooked)

1/2 cup celery (diced)

1/2 cup raw walnuts (chopped) or raw almonds (slivered)

2 tsp lemon juice or apple cider vinegar

2/3 cup Veganaise (or mayo with no bad oil)

Salt and pepper (to taste)

Optional add-ins: granny smith apple, grapes, dried cranberries, raisins, other nuts, etc.

Spinach or wraps (for serving - optional)

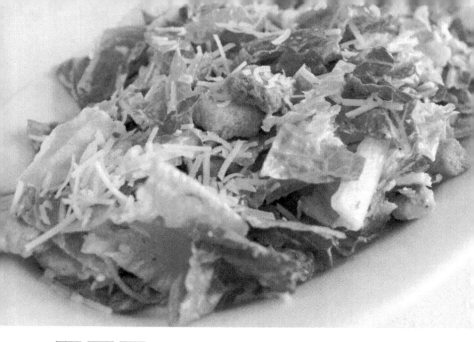

Caesar Salad
Serves 2 | 30 Minutes

2 organic chicken breasts
(cooked how desired)

Organic spinach and romaine
lettuce

Dressing:
1/2 cup olive oil

1 lemon (juiced, can add zest
as well)

1/3 cup organic parmesan
cheese

4 tsp dijon mustard

2 garlic cloves or garlic
powder

1 tbsp worcestershire sauce,
more or less (to taste)

Salt and pepper (to taste)

Mix or blend all dressing ingredients together until smooth. Combine chicken, spinach, romaine and dressing in a bowl with a lid and shake until completely covered. Add more parmesan cheese to top before eating.

Anti-Inflammatory Plan Tip:
Avoid cheese.

Vegetarian Plan Tip:
Approved for vegetarians that eat eggs and/or dairy. Remove chicken.

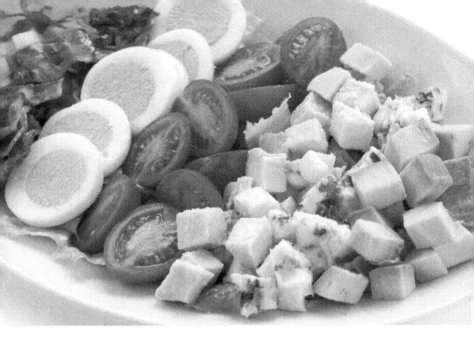

Cobb Salad

Serves 2 | 30 Minutes

I bake or boil my chicken to get it cooked quickly! You can also grill it for added flavor. Cook the turkey bacon and make your hard-boiled eggs (boil eggs in water for approximately 10 minutes). Cut the cooked chicken breast in slices and put over a bed of spinach. Add blue cheese crumbles and toppings that you like. Pour over the ranch dressing and toss until coated.

2 organic chicken breasts
(cooked how desired)

1/2 cup turkey bacon
(pre-cooked)

2 organic eggs (hard-boiled)

4 cups spinach

1/4 cup blue cheese crumbles

1/4-1/2 cup Homemade Ranch Dressing Recipe (see recipe page 165)

Optional toppings: cucumber, tomato, carrot, celery, avocado, red onion

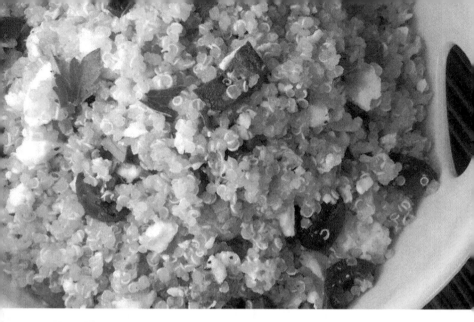

Mediterranean Quinoa Salad
Serves 4 | 20 Minutes + 30 Minutes Chill Time

1 cup quinoa (uncooked) or spinach (for serving)

2 limes (zest and juice)

4 oz feta cheese (crumbed)

2 oz kalamata olives (chopped, with brine)

1/4 cup fresh parsley (chopped)

Pepper (to taste)

Cucumbers (optional)

Cook the quinoa according to package directions. Remove from heat and let cool briefly. Stir the lime zest, lime juice, feta cheese, chopped olives, and fresh parsley into the quinoa until thoroughly mixed. Season with pepper, if desired. Refrigerate for at least 30 minutes before serving for more flavor.

Anti-Inflammatory Plan Tip: Avoid cheese.

Low Carb Plan Tip: Ideal to not eat quinoa on the low carb plan. You could make a Mediterranean salad by putting cooked chicken and the rest of the ingredients on a salad. Try adding cucumbers too!

Vegetarian Plan Tip: Approved for vegetarians that eat eggs and/or dairy.

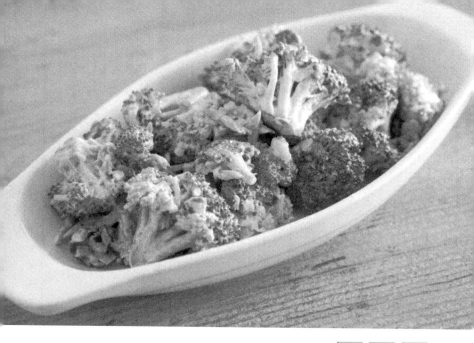

Easy Broccoli Salad

Serves 4 | 20 Minutes + 1 Hour Chill Time

In a large bowl, mix together the mayo, vinegar, and sweetener. Add in the rest of the ingredients and stir until coated completely. Add more or less "sauce" as desired. Refrigerate for an hour before serving for best flavor and toss once more before eating.

Anti-Inflammatory Plan Tip:
Avoid the peppers. Nuts and seeds are options for this plan, in moderation, if no known sensitivities.

Low Carb Plan Tip:
Avoid the dried fruit.

Vegetarian Plan Tip:
Approved for vegetarians that eat eggs and/or dairy.

1 cup Veganaise or Primal Kitchen Avocado Oil Mayo

2 tbsp apple cider vinegar

1 tbsp sweetener (i.e. Swerve)

2 heads broccoli (cut into florets)

1 cup mixed bell peppers (diced)

1/8 cup red onion (diced tiny)

1/4 cup dried cranberries or raisins

1/4 cup nuts or seeds, (chopped if necessary - almonds, walnuts, sunflower seeds, etc.)

Optional: add slivered brussels sprouts, carrots, or cabbage for added nutrients

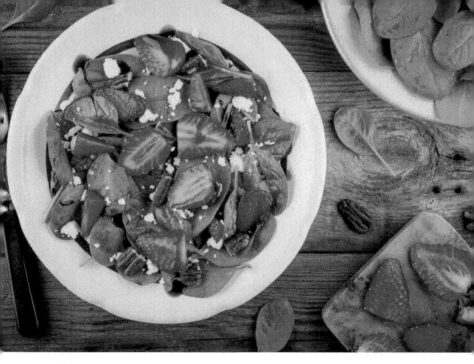

   ## Strawberry Goat Cheese Salad

Serves 1 | 15 Minutes

2 cups organic spinach

1 cup organic strawberries (sliced)

1/2 cup raw pecans (or use Candied Pecan Recipe)

1/2 cup goat cheese (crumbles)

Dressing (your choice of): Oil and vinegar, balsamic vinegar (i.e. Primal Kitchen, Bragg's Brand, Tessemae Brand)

Optional toppings: grilled chicken, grilled salmon, cucumber, tomatoes, red onion, slivered almonds, dates, figs, avocado

Take any of the ingredients listed, as much as desired, and make a delicious, quick and easy salad. So light and refreshing.

Anti-Inflammatory Plan Tip: Nuts are options for this plan, in moderation, if no known sensitivities. Avoid the cheese all together.

Vegetarian Plan Tip: Approved for vegetarians that eat eggs and/or dairy.

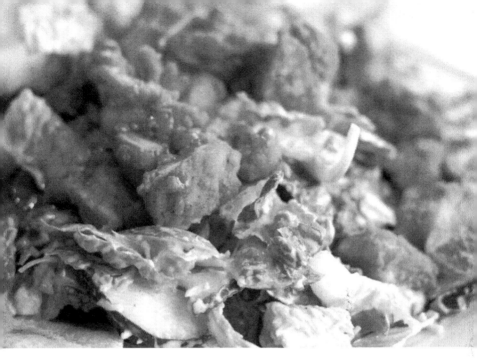

Buffalo Chicken Salad

Serves 2 | 1 Hour

Pour the buffalo or hot sauce over the chicken breasts and bake at 350 degrees F for approximately one hour. When the chicken is almost done you can put some blue cheese crumbles on top to melt over the chicken. Cut the cooked chicken breast in slices and put over a bed of spinach. Add any additional blue cheese crumbles and toppings that you like. We like to pour over the ranch dressing and a little more hot sauce!

Slow Cooker Option:
You can put the chicken and sauce in a crock pot if you prefer (2-3 hours on high, 4-5 hours on low).

You can also make DLG's Boneless Wings Recipe and put the wings on top of a salad.

2 organic chicken breasts

1/2 cup buffalo sauce or hot sauce (Tessemee is a great brand)

1/4 cup blue cheese crumbles

3 cups organic spinach

1/4-1/2 cup Homemade Ranch Dressing (see recipe page 165)

Optional toppings: cucumber, tomato, carrot, celery, avocado, red onion

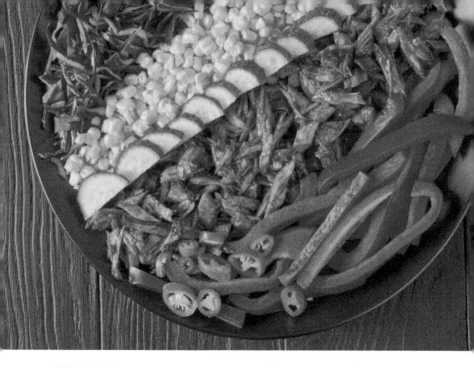

BBQ Chicken Salad

Serves 2 | 30 Minutes

2 chicken breasts (cooked how desired)

1 cup BBQ Sauce

4 cups spinach

1/4 cup organic cheddar cheese (shredded)

1/2 cup cabbage (shredded)

1/2 cup cucumbers (diced)

1/2 cup organic non-GMO corn (optional)

1/2 cup red bell peppers (diced)

1/4 cup tomatoes (diced)

1/4-1/2 cup Homemade Ranch Dressing (see recipe page 165)

Bake the chicken until cooked through. You can also grill it for added flavor. Shred the cooked chicken breast and mix well with the BBQ sauce (add more if desired). Put over a bed of spinach or put into your wrap of choice. Add cheese, toppings, and ranch dressing and toss until coated if making a salad.

Slow Cooker Option: You can also add chicken in a slow cooker with the BBQ sauce and cook slowly on low heat for 4-6 hours

Anti-Inflammatory Plan Tip: Watch ingredients in the BBQ sauce. Avoid cheese and peppers all together. Tomatos are an option for this plan, in moderation, if no known sensitivities. Also, avoid egg-based dressings.

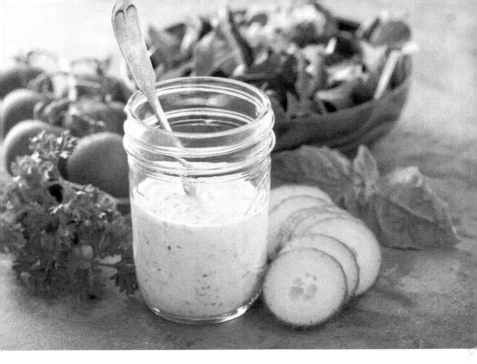

Homemade Ranch Dressing

Yields 1 1/4 Cups Of Dressing | 15 Minutes + 1-2 Hours Chill Time

Put all ingredients in a high-powered blender or food processor and blend well until smooth consistency. Refrigerate 1-2 hours for best results. Enjoy within a week.

Low Carb Plan Tip:
Watch the ingredients in the mayos – they like to hide sugar in them!

Vegetarian Plan Tip:
Approved for vegetarians that eat eggs and/or dairy.

1 cup mayonnaise (watch ingredients. Primal Kitchen brand, Chosen Foods brand with Avocado oil or soy free Vegenaise are good options)

1/2 cup fresh parsley

1/4 cup lemon (juice + zest)

2-3 garlic cloves (or use garlic powder)

1-2 tbsp fresh dill or dried dill (to taste)

1/2 tsp sea salt

Pepper (to taste)

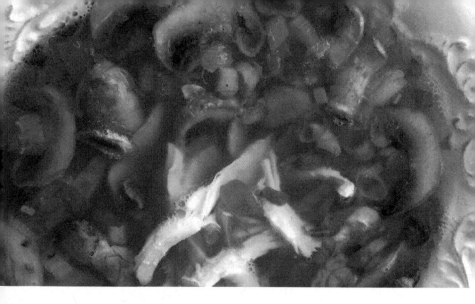

Chicken Marsala Soup

Serves 6 | 25 Minutes

3 tbsp extra virgin olive oil

8 oz white mushrooms (sliced)

Sea salt and pepper (to taste)

4 green onions (ends removed and chopped thin, white and green parts separated)

2/3 cup dry marsala wine

6 cups organic chicken or vegetable broth

2 organic chicken breasts (cooked and diced)

Over medium heat in a large sauce or soup pan, add olive oil and mushrooms and cook. Continue cooking for approximately 5 minutes until mushrooms start to release their juices, stirring occasionally. Season with salt and pepper, to taste. Add white parts of onion to pan and cook for 1-2 minutes, stirring once or twice. Increase heat to high and add the marsala wine. Cook until wine has reduced to 1/3 of its volume, approximately 5 minutes. Add chicken broth and cooked chicken and bring to a boil. Reduce heat to just below medium. Simmer until heated through, approximately 5 minutes. Remove from heat and serve. Garnish with green parts of onion.

Vegetarian Plan Tip: Replace chicken with diced cauliflower florets.

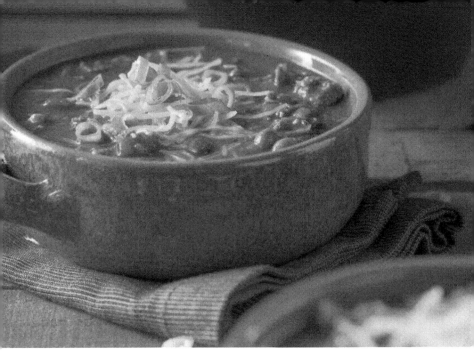

Simple Chili

Serves 4 | 30 Minutes

Brown beef in a large pot until cooked. Add all other ingredients and simmer until beans are soft. Add toppings as desired

Slow Cooker Option:
You can also leave all ingredients in a slow cooker for 3-4 hours on low.

Anti-Inflammatory Plan Tip:
Tomatos and beans are options for this plan, in moderation, if no known sensitivities. Avoid optional toppings and chili powder.

Vegetarian Plan Tip:
Remove meat for an all bean chili.

1 lb grass-fed beef or bison

1 onion (diced)

1 large can tomatoes (diced)

1 small can tomato sauce

2 cans kidney beans

1 can black beans

2 tbsp chili powder

3 tbsp cumin

Salt, pepper, garlic powder, cayenne pepper (to taste)

Optional toppings: organic sour cream, chives, organic cheese

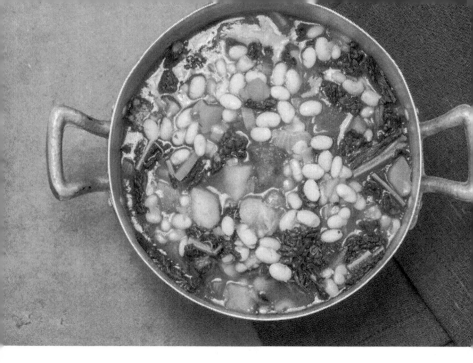

Vegetable and Bean Soup
Serves 6 | 60 Minutes

4 stalks of celery (diced)

1/2 cup of parsley (can also add other spices like sage, if desired)

1 yellow squash (diced)

1 zucchini (diced)

2 cloves of garlic (minced)

6 cups of chicken bone broth or vegetable broth

2 cups cabbage (purple or green)

2 cups kale (chopped)

2 cans of cannellini beans (drained and rinsed)

Salt and pepper (to taste)

Sauté all of the vegetables and seasonings in oil (except kale and cabbage) in large stock pot for about 10-15 minutes. Add broth and the rest of the ingredients to the pot and allow to simmer for 30-40 minutes. Add salt and pepper to taste.

Anti-Inflammatory Plan Tip: Beans are options for this plan, in moderation, if no known sensitivities.

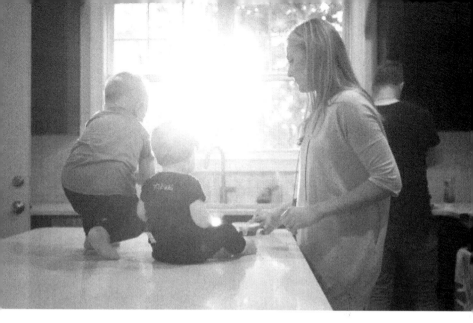

DESSERTS

Almond Butter Cups · 170

Chocolate Chip Cookies · 171

Lemon Pound Cake · 172

DLG Favorite Chia Seed Pudding · 173

Peanut Butter Cookies · 174

Cinnamon Ice Cream · 175

Ginger Cookies · 176

Mini Cheesecakes · 177

Almond Cookies · 178

Black Bean Brownies · 179

Berry Cobbler · 180

Pumpkin Spice Brownies · 181

Simple Frosting · 182

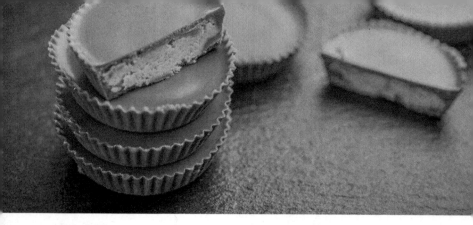

Almond Butter Cups
Yields 6-8 Cups | 25 Minutes

Chocolate:
1/4 cup butter

4-6 tbsp of coconut oil

2 tsp vanilla extract

2 bars of unsweetened chocolate bars

Stevia (to taste - liquid or powder - NOW brand, KAL brand stevias or Swerve are good - probably need more than you are expecting to take away bitter flavor)

Sea salt (to taste)

Filling:
Raw almond butter or nut butter of choice (watch for bad oils)

Toppings (optional):
Whole raw almonds, pecans, walnuts

In a saucepan, melt butter, coconut oil, vanilla, and chocolate squares over low heat. Remove from heat. Add stevia or sweetener of choice. Line muffin tin with paper liners and put approximately 2 spoonfuls of melted chocolate to cover just the bottom of paper/tin. Put in freezer for a few minutes until "set" or firm. Once removed, scoop as much almond butter into each cup, as desired. Approximately 1 tbsp. Cover nut butter with chocolate until and smooth on top. Sprinkle sea salt on top. Put in freezer until completely set. Keep in freezer until ready to eat for best results.

*If no muffin pan, use parchment paper on bottom of a cookie sheet or cake pan and make "bark" type of chocolates with nuts. Or, in desperate situations, you can also use a plastic egg carton in place of a muffin pan. ;)

Vegetarian Plan Tip:
Approved for vegetarians that eat eggs and/or dairy.

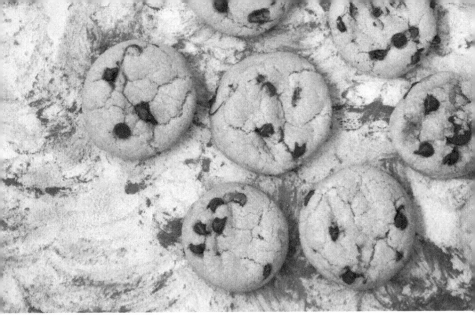

Chocolate Chip Cookies

Yields 12 Cookies | 20 Minutes

In a bowl, combine all ingredients except the chocolate chips and mix until a creamy batter is made. Stir in chocolate chips. Make into cookie balls and place on an unbleached parchment paper lined baking sheet. Put in the oven for approximately 5 minutes. Flatten the cookies to desired thickness (cookies will not rise much and do not spread). Bake for approximately 10 more minutes, or until golden brown, at 350 degrees F.

Low Carb Plan Tip:
Remove the sweetener (honey/maple syrup) and try coconut sugar, xylitol, stevia, or Swerve, to taste. These substitutes may make cookies dry so might add more oil or egg if so

Vegetarian Plan Tip:
Approved for vegetarians that eat eggs and/or dairy.

2 organic eggs

3 cups almond flour

1 tsp vanilla extract

4 tbsp coconut oil (softened)

1/4 cup maple syrup

1/2 tsp baking soda

1/2 tsp sea salt

1 cup stevia-sweetened chocolate chips

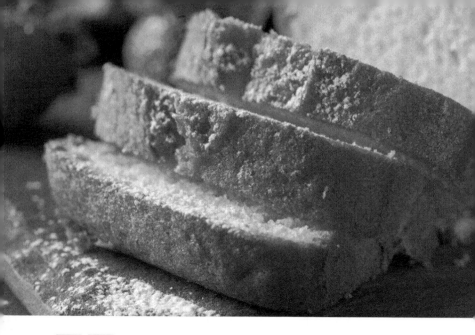

Lemon Pound Cake
Serves 8 | 30 Minutes

1 stick butter

1/2 cup xylitol or Swerve

4 organic eggs

1/2 tbsp lemon extract (if no lemon flavor use one tbsp vanilla extract)

1 tsp baking powder

2 cups almond flour

Coconut oil or butter (for greasing)

Optional Whipped Cream Topping:
1 can coconut milk

1 tsp vanilla

Swerve or Swerve Confectioners' Sugar Substitute, to taste

Fresh berries

Cream butter & xylitol together until smooth. Add in one egg at a time until fluffy. Add lemon extract or flavor and baking powder. Once blended add the almond flour until smooth. Grease a loaf pan with coconut oil or butter and bake at 350 degrees F for approximately 45 minutes or until golden brown.

To make whipped coconut milk, combine coconut milk and Swerve and mix with hand mixer until the coconut milk is stiff and forms peaks. Chill and pull out when ready to eat and add fresh berries.

Vegetarian Plan Tip:
Approved for vegetarians that eat eggs and/or dairy.

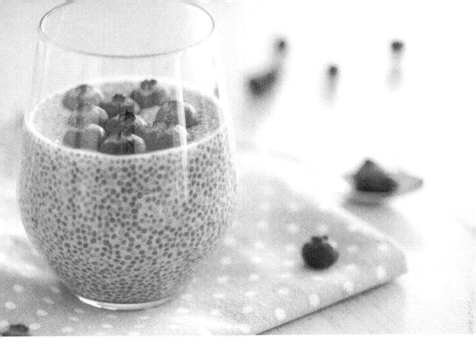

DLG Favorite Chia Seed Pudding

Serves 4 | 5 Minutes + 2 Hours Chill Time

Put all ingredients in a blender and blend on high for 1-2 minutes until smooth. If you prefer the chia seeds not to be blended, just stir until well mixed. Pour into a container and refrigerate for minimum of 2-3 hours up to overnight. Top with your favorite toppings and enjoy! Best if eaten within a couple of days.

Anti-Inflammatory Plan Tip:
Coconut, almond, cashew, and flax milk are options for this plan as well as chocolate and cacao, in moderation, if no known sensitivities.

Low Carb Plan Tip:
Remove the sweetener (honey, maple syrup, etc.) and use more Livingood Daily Chocolate Greens or Collagen Protein.

Vegetarian Plan Tip:
Approved for vegetarians that eat eggs and/or dairy.

1 can coconut milk

1/2 cup chia seeds

1/2 tsp vanilla extract

1 scoop Livingood Daily Vanilla or Chocolate Collagen Protein

Cinnamon (to taste - optional)

1/2 scoop Livingood Daily Chocolate Greens (optional)

1 tbsp maple syrup (optional)

Toppings (optional):
Berries, chopped nuts, unsweetened coconut flakes, cacao nibs

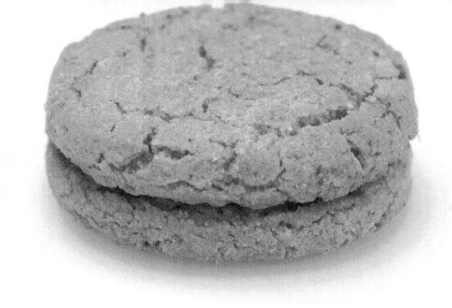

Peanut Butter Cookie

Yields 1 Dozen | 25 Minutes

1 organic egg

1 tsp vanilla extract

1/4 cup honey

3/4 cup almond butter or organic valencia peanut butter

2 tbsp coconut sugar (or sub 2 tbsp additional honey in place)

3/4 cup almond flour

1/4 tsp sea salt

2 dashes nutmeg

1/4 tsp cinnamon

1/4 tsp baking soda

Optional: stevia sweetened chocolate chips

Whisk together egg, vanilla extract and honey. Add in nut butter and mix thoroughly. Fold in dry ingredients and mix again. Using a cookie scoop or two spoons, divide dough into a dozen cookies and place on a parchment paper covered baking sheet. Bake for 14 minutes at 325 degrees F.

Low Carb Plan Tip: Remove the sweetener (honey/maple syrup) and try coconut sugar, xylitol, or stevia, to taste.

Vegetarian Plan Tip: Approved for vegetarians that eat eggs and/or dairy.

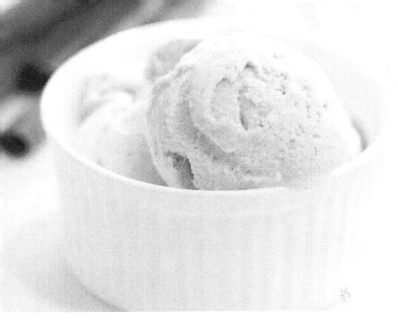

Cinnamon Ice Cream

Serves 2-4 | 15 Minutes + Chill Time

Put all ingredients into a high-powered blender and blend until smooth consistency. Pour the blended mixture into an ice cream maker*. Follow the instructions on the ice cream maker.

*If you don't own an ice cream maker, you can add chilled mixture to a freezer-safe container and freeze. Once every hour, remove from freezer and stir/whisk to incorporate air. Repeat until mostly firm (6-8 hours). Then continue freezing until completely firm before serving. The results won't be quite as creamy, but it will still work!

Low Carb Plan Tip:
Avoid maple syrup and try Livingood Daily Collagen Protein.

Vegetarian Plan Tip:
Approved for vegetarians that eat eggs and/or dairy.

2 cans coconut milk or coconut cream

2 tbsp butter (melted)

3 tsp cinnamon

2 tsp vanilla extract

1/4 tsp sea salt

1/4 cup maple syrup (or you can use 2 droppers full of liquid stevia or 1/4 cup coconut sugar or 1/4 cup almond butter)

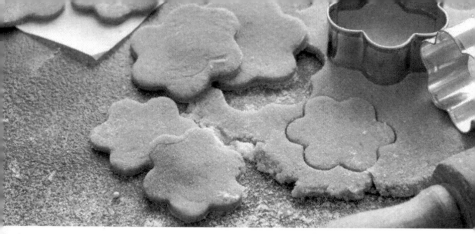

Gingerbread Cookies

Yields 12-15 Cookies | 30 Minutes

3 cups almond flour

1/2 cup arrowroot or tapioca starch (extra for rolling and cutting)

4 tsp ground ginger

1 tsp ground cinnamon

1/4 tsp sea salt

1/2 tsp baking soda

4 tbsp coconut oil (melted)

1/4-1/2 cup maple syrup

2 tbsp molasses

Simple Frosting (see recipe page 182 - optional)

In a large bowl, mix all dry ingredients well. Add in the coconut oil, maple syrup and the molasses and stir until a sticky dough is formed. Place the dough in the freezer for 30 minutes to help it be less sticky. Once chilled, place the dough on parchment paper that is sprinkled with a little arrowroot or tapioca starch to prevent sticking. Use a rolling pan (or your hands) and flatten the dough until about 1/4 -inch thick. Use your cookie cutters and cut your cookies. With the excess dough, re-roll and cut more out until you have no dough remaining. You can also just roll the dough into cookie balls and flatten them out with your hand to make circles if you don't have cookie cutters. Bake the cookies at 350 degrees F for approximately 10-12 minutes. Frost with simple frosting recipe, if desired.

Anti-Inflammatory Plan Tip: Coconut flour, almond flour, cassava flour and flax meal are options for this plan, in moderation, if no known sensitivities.

Low Carb Plan Tip: Remove the sweetener (honey/maple syrup) and try coconut sugar, xylitol, or stevia, to taste.

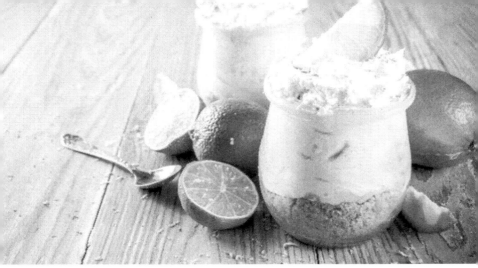

Mini Cheesecakes

Yields 6 Muffin-Sized | 25 Minutes + 4 Hours Chill Time

Soak cashews in filtered water overnight.

Crust:
Mix almonds and coconut oil in a food processor until mixture is crumbly but sticks together when forming. Place 2-3 tbsp of crust in a lined muffin cup (6 muffins) and press down to form the crust bottom. Place muffin tin in the freezer to set for approximately 15 minutes.

Topping:
Combine the drained cashews, coconut oil, coconut milk, stevia, lime juice and most of the zest in a high-powered blender or food processor. Mix until smooth. Add more stevia if needed. Pour the mixture into the muffin tins over the crust. Sprinkle the extra lime zest on top and chill in the refrigerator for approximately 4-6 hours or until hardened. Best if kept chilled.

Anti-Inflammatory Plan Tip:
Coconut oil and milk are options for this plan as well as nuts, in moderation, if no known sensitivities.

Crust:
1 cup almonds

1/4 cup coconut oil (melted)

Topping:
1 cup cashews (soaked in hot water overnight, drained)

1/2 cup coconut oil (melted)

1 can coconut milk (mixed well)

1 tsp liquid stevia (to taste - or sweetener like Swerve)

4 limes (juiced and zested)

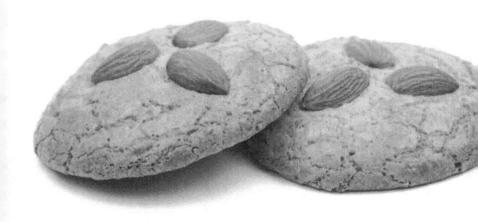

Almond Cookies

Yields 10 Cookies | 25 Minutes

2 cups almond flour

2 organic eggs

1 tbsp almond extract

1/4 tsp sea salt

1/2 tsp baking soda

1 tbsp coconut oil (melted)

1/2 tsp fresh grated lemon zest or few drops lemon extract

2 tbsp spoonable stevia or Swerve

Slivered almonds (topping - optional)

Mix together all ingredients. Shape into small balls and place on parchment paper lined baking sheet. Bake at 350 degrees F for approximately 15 minutes or until golden brown. Can top with slivered almonds if desire.

Vegetarian Plan Tip:
Approved for vegetarians that eat eggs and/or dairy.

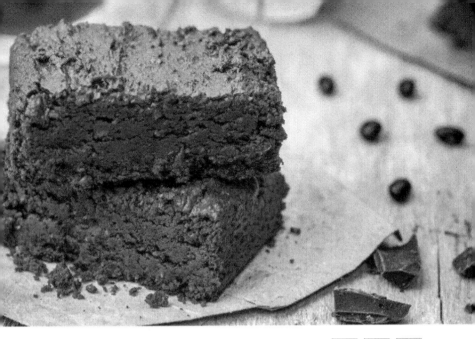

Black Bean Brownies

Yields 12 | 40 Minutes

Combine all ingredients, except chocolate chips, in a food processor or use a hand mixer and mix until completely smooth. Stir in the chocolate chips. Using coconut oil lightly grease the bottom of an 8 8 baking dish. Pour the batter into the baking dish and sprinkle with more chocolate chips, if desired, for appearance. Bake for approximately 30-35 minutes on 350 degrees F. Let cool 10 minutes before cutting and serving.

Anti-Inflammatory Plan Tip: Coconut flour and flax meal are options for this plan as well as cacao, in moderation, if no known sensitivities.

Low Carb Plan Tip: Remove the sweetener (honey/maple syrup) and try coconut sugar, xylitol, or stevia, to taste.

1-15oz can black beans (rinsed well)

4 tbsp cocoa powder

1/2 cup quick oats, flax meal, or paleo flour

1/4 tsp salt

1/3 cup maple syrup or honey

2 tbsp coconut sugar (or Swerve)

1/4 cup coconut oil (melted)

2 tsp vanilla extract

1/2 tsp baking powder

1/2 cup stevia-sweetened chocolate chips

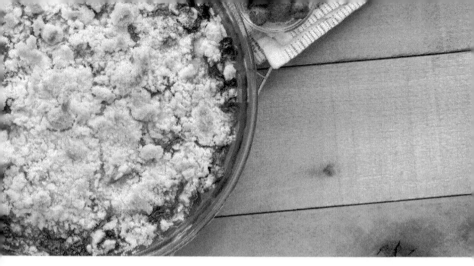

Berry Cobbler

Serves 9-12 | 90 Minutes

Crust:
2 cups almond flour

1/4 cup coconut oil

1/4 cup maple syrup

1/8 tsp sea salt

Fruit and Jam Center:
4 cups frozen or fresh berries
(finely cut - can do all of the
same or mix it up)

1/4 cup maple syrup

2 tbsp arrowroot powder

Crumb Topping:
1 cup almond flour

2 tbsp coconut oil

2 tbsp maple syrup

Pinch of sea salt

In a large bowl, mix all of the crust ingredients with a mixer. Evenly press the dough into an 8 8 inch-baking pan lined with parchment paper. Bake at 350 degrees F for 15 minutes. Mix the center fruit and jam ingredients in a medium-sized pot and turn on low heat. Continue stirring the ingredients until the mixture has thickened. After about 20 minutes, when the consistency is similar to jam, remove from heat. Spread the filling over the baked crust. Mix crumb topping with hand mixer in a medium-sized bowl. Sprinkle the crumb topping over the filling. Bake for 35-40 minutes or until the crumbles are lightly brown. Allow to cool for approximately 10-15 minutes before serving. Store in the refrigerator and can serve cool.

Anti-Inflammatory Plan Tip:
Coconut flour, almond flour, arrowroot (cassava flour) and flax meal are options for this plan, in moderation, if no known sensitivities.

Low Carb Plan Tip:
Remove the sweetener (honey/maple syrup) and try coconut sugar, xylitol, or stevia, to taste.

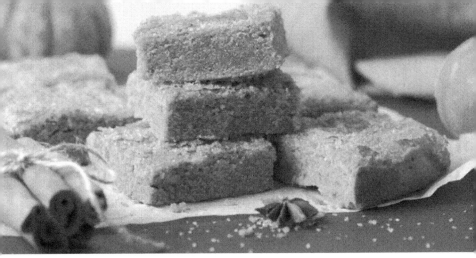

Pumpkin Spice "Brownie"

Yields 9-12 | 45 Minutes

Combine all ingredients, except chocolate chips, in a food processor or use a hand mixer and mix until completely smooth. Stir in the chocolate chips. Using coconut oil lightly grease the bottom of an 8 8 baking dish. Pour the batter into the baking dish and sprinkle with more chocolate chips, if desired, for appearance. Bake for approximately 25-30 minutes on 350 degrees F. Let cool 10 minutes before cutting and serving. Top with Simple Frosting, if desired.

Anti-Inflammatory Plan Tip:
Coconut flour, almond flour, cassava flour and flax meal are options for this plan, in moderation, if no known sensitivities.

Low Carb Plan Tip:
Remove the sweetener (honey/ maple syrup) and try coconut sugar, xylitol, or stevia, to taste.

1/4 cup coconut flour

1/4 cup almond flour

1/4 cup tapioca starch or arrowroot

1/4-1/2 cup coconut sugar (can use other sweeteners if you prefer – Swerve)

1/4 tsp baking powder

1/2 tsp baking soda

1 cup canned organic pumpkin

3/4 cup almond butter

1/4 cup maple syrup (or honey)

3 tsp pumpkin spice

2 tsp cinnamon

1 tsp sea salt

Coconut oil (for greasing)

Stevia-sweetened chocolate chips (optional topping)

Simple Frosting (see recipe page 182 - optional)

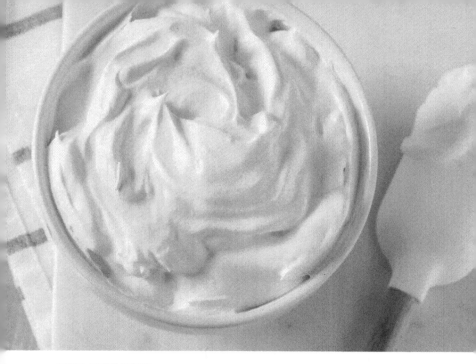

Simple Frosting

Yields 1 Cup | 15 Minutes

6 tbsp coconut butter (or organic butter) (melted)

1 tsp vanilla extract

2 tbsp (+) Swerve Confectioners Sweetener

4-6 tbsp almond milk (or other non-dairy milk or choice or organic heavy cream)

Slowly melt the coconut butter on low heat. Remove from the heat and add vanilla and sweetener. Add the milk one tablespoon at a time, stirring in between until a smooth, frosting-like consistency.

We recommend using this simple frosting for the Gingerbread Cookies (page 176) or on top of the Pumpkin Spice Brownies (page 181).

Anti-Inflammatory Plan Tip: Coconut butter and almond milk are options for this plan, in moderation, if no known sensitivities.

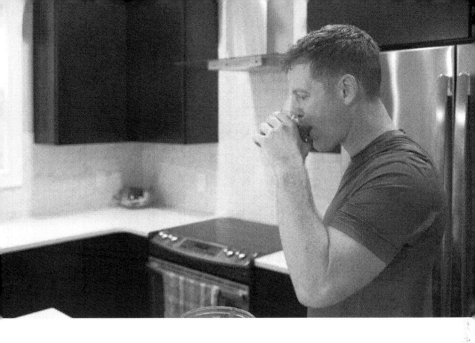

DRINKS

Immune Boosting Green Juice   184

Bulletproof Matcha Latte   185

Quick Homemade Lemonade or Limeade   186

Anti-Inflammatory Beet Juice   187

Chia Latte   188

DLG Pumpkin Spice Latte   189

Healthy Hot Chocolate   190

DLG Bulletproof Coffee   191

DLG Apple Cidar Vinegar Drink   192

Jalapeno Cucumber Lemonade   193

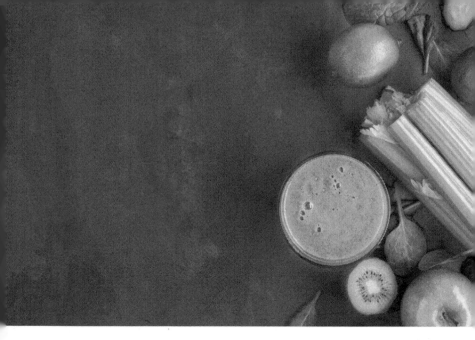

   Immune Boosting Green Juice

Serves 1 | 10 Minutes

4-6 celery stalks

1 cucumber (skin off)

1 granny smith apple

2 cups spinach and/or kale

1 head of romaine lettuce

1 lemon*

1 lime (optional)

1 small knob ginger (optional)

Juice all ingredients in a juicer. Stir and serve over ice if desired!

*Depending on juicer, you may need to peel the lemon but leave as much of the white pith on as you can.

If you do not have a juicer, you can also put everything in a blender on high. Pour into a fine mesh strainer or through a nut milk bag for a less pulpy, silky smooth result.

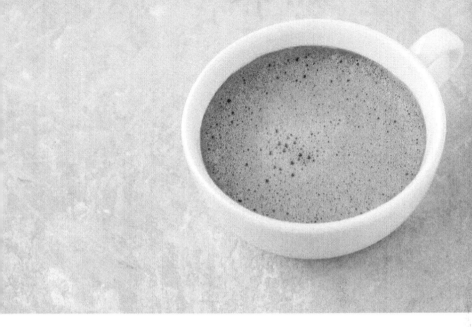

Bulletproof Matcha Latte

Serves 1 | 5 Minutes

Bring the water and nut milk to a boil (or you can just use 1 1/2 cups of nut milk instead of water). Put all ingredients into a blender and blend on high until smooth and frothy!

Anti-Inflammatory Plan Tip:
Nut milks are options for this plan, in moderation, if no known sensitivities.

Vegetarian Plan Tip:
Remove Collagen Protein. Add stevia, for taste.

1/2 cup of water

1 cup unsweetened nut milk

1 1/2 tsp organic matcha powder

1/2 scoop Livingood Daily Vanilla Collagen Protein

1 tbsp coconut oil

1 tbsp ghee or butter

1 tsp sea salt

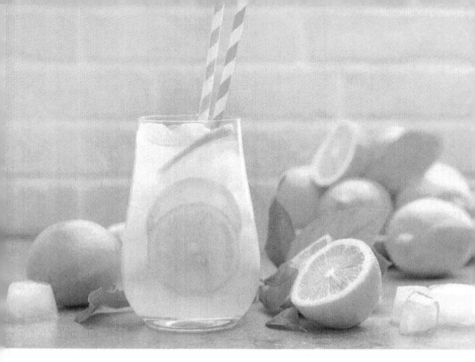

Quick Homemade Lemonade or Limeade

Serves 1 | 10 Minutes

2 cups of water

1 fresh squeezed lemon

1 fresh squeezed lime

10-12 drops liquid stevia (to taste - can substitute xylitol or Swerve)

Ice

Added fun: try half water, half sparkling water or adding fresh mint

Stir all ingredients until mixed well and serve over ice. Add more or less stevia as desired.

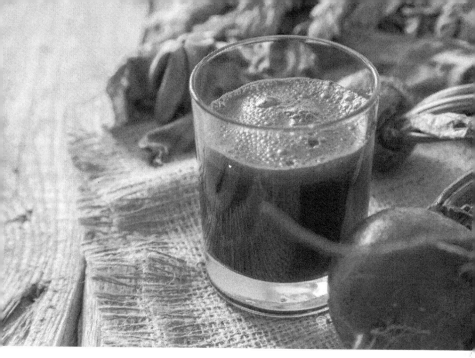

Anti-Inflammatory Beet Juice

Serves 1 | 10 Minutes

Cut all pieces into sizes that will fit into your juicer. Put all ingredients in your juicer and enjoy!

*Depending on juicer, you may need to peel the lemon but leave as much of the white pith on as you can.

If you do not have a juicer, you can also put everything in a blender on high. Pour into a fine mesh strainer or through a nut milk bag for a less pulpy, silky smooth result.

1 granny smith apple

1 medium beet root (peeled)

1/2 cucumber (peeled)

6 stalks of celery

1 small ginger root (approx. 1")

1 tsp fresh turmeric

1/2-1 lemon*

Optional: carrots, leafy greens, parsley

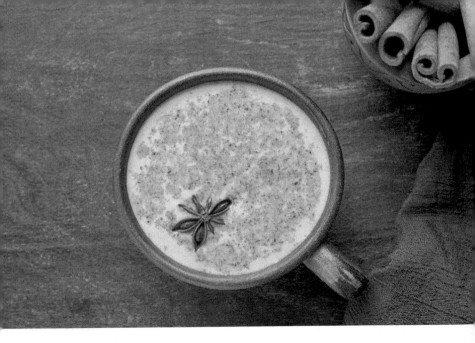

Chai Latte

Serves 1 | 10 Minutes

1 1/2 cups almond or coconut milk

2 organic chai tea bags

Cinnamon (to taste)

Option 2 - If not using tea bags:
1 tsp cinnamon

1/4 tsp ginger

1/8 tsp cloves

1 tbsp maple syrup (or sweetener of choice)

In a small saucepan over medium/high heat, bring the milk to a boil while steeping the chai tea bags for approximately 5 minutes. Or if using spices whisk together and heat until boiling hot.

Anti-Inflammatory Plan Tip: Coconut, almond, cashew, and flax milk are options for this plan, in moderation, if no known sensitivities.

Low Carb Plan Tip: Remove the sweetener (honey/maple syrup) and try coconut sugar, xylitol, or stevia, to taste.

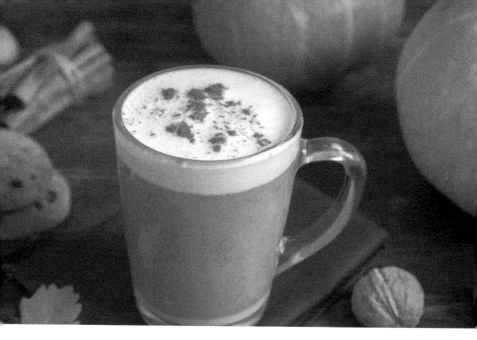

DLG Pumpkin Spice Latte

Serves 1 | 10 Minutes

Heat the coconut milk on the stove. Add all ingredients into a blender and blend until smooth. Pour into a mug and sprinkle with pumpkin spice, if desired.

*Can make homemade whipped cream topping with just the fat from the coconut milk. Chill it and blend on high until creamed.

Anti-Inflammatory Plan Tip: Coconut, almond, cashew, flax milk, and coffee are options for this plan, in moderation, if no known sensitivities.

Low Carb Plan Tip: Remove the sweetener (honey/ maple syrup) and try coconut sugar, xylitol, or stevia, to taste.

1 cup coconut milk

1/2 cup strong organic coffee (or 1/4 cup espresso)

2 tbsp organic pumpkin puree

1 scoop of Livingood Daily Vanilla Collagen Protein

1 tbsp maple syrup (optional)

1/2 tsp vanilla extract

1/2 tsp pumpkin spice

Coconut cream or fat from coconut milk when chilled (optional)

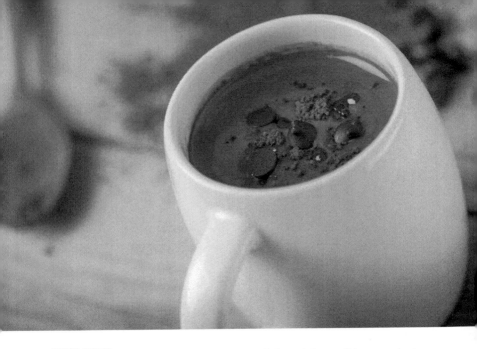

Healthy Hot Chocolate

Serves 1 | 10 Minutes

1 cup unsweetened almond milk or coconut milk

2 tbsp cacao powder

2 ounces cocoa bar (optional)

1 tbsp maple syrup

1 tsp vanilla extract

1 pinch sea salt

1/2 scoop Livingood Daily Chocolate Collagen Protein or Chocolate Greens (optional)

*Coconut cream or fat from coconut milk when chilled (optional)

Combine all the ingredients into a saucepan over high heat, using a whisk to break up any clumps. Stir until smooth and hot, then pour into a mug and enjoy.

*Can make homemade whipped cream topping with just the fat from coconut milk. Chill it and blend on high until creamed.

Low Carb Plan Tip: Remove the sweetener (honey/maple syrup) and try liquid stevia, to taste.

Vegetarian Plan Tip: Approved for vegetarians that eat eggs and/or dairy.

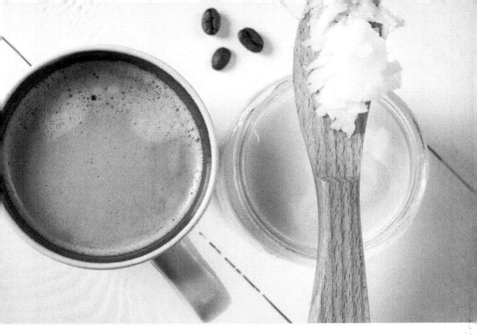

DLG Bulletproof Coffee

Serves 1 | 10 Minutes

Put everything into a blender and blend until it's frothy. Pour into a cup and sprinkle with cinnamon.

Anti-Inflammatory Plan Tip:
Coconut oil is an option for this plan as well as coffee, in moderation, if no known sensitivities. Remove the butter.

12-16oz organic coffee

1 tbsp coconut oil

1 tbsp butter

1/4 scoop Livingood Daily Vanilla Collagen Protein

1/4 tsp cinnamon powder (topping)

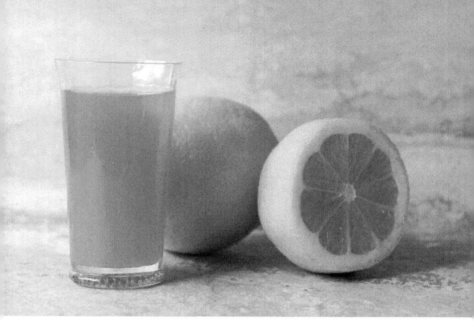

   DLG Apple Cidar Vinegar Drink

Serves 1 | 5 Minutes

2 tsp Dr. Livingood High
Dose Vitamin C

1 tsp Probiotic Powder

1 tbsp apple cider vinegar

12 oz water or sparkling
water

Put all ingredients into a cup and stir
until well mixed. Add ice if you prefer
a chilled drink. Enjoy!

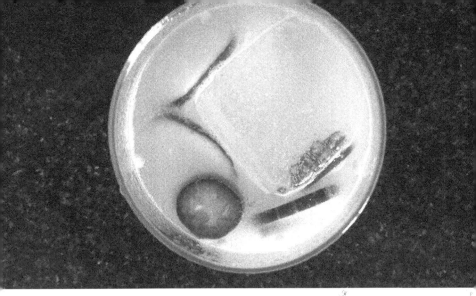

Jalapeno Cucumber Lemonade

Serves 4-6 | 15 Minutes

You can either juice all ingredients in a juicer or add water, lemon juice, cucumber, jalapeno, and honey to a blender and blend until completely liquefied. Taste and add more jalapeno and/or sweetener, if desired. Blend again if necessary. If you blend, you can pour liquid through a fine mesh strainer to remove any larger particles. Transfer to a large pitcher and place in refrigerator to chill for at least 1 hour before serving. Pour over ice and garnish with optional garnishes.

Low Carb Plan Tip:
Remove the sweetener (honey/maple syrup) and try coconut sugar, xylitol, or stevia, to taste.

3 cups of water

3/4 cups fresh lemon juice (6-8 lemons)

1 large cucumber (peeled and cut into chunks)

2 tsp jalapeno pepper, seeds removed (finely minced)

1/4 cup honey

Optional garnishes:
Rosemary sprigs with lower leaves removed, cucumber chunks or slices, jalapeno chunks or slices, lemon wedges

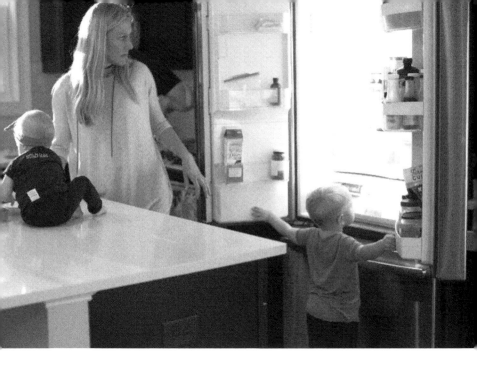

SNACKS

Homemade Hummus Dip   196

Energy Cookie Balls   197

Cinnamon Baked Nuts   198

Candied Nuts   199

Make Your Own Trail Mix   200

Guacamole   201

Green Apple Snacks   202

Sweet Potato Chips   203

Popsicles   204

Fruit Honey-Yogurt Dip   206

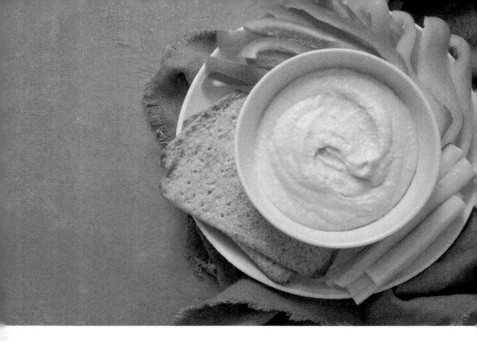

Homemade Hummus Dip

Yields 1 Cup | 15 Minutes

1-15 oz can chickpeas

2 tbsp olive oil

1 juice of a lemon

1/4 cup tahini

1 tbsp cumin (to taste)

1 tsp sea salt (to taste)

1 tsp paprika (optional)

Optional flavors:
- 1 clove garlic
- 2 fire roasted red peppers
- jalepeno and cilantro
- or sub chickpeas for black beans

Drain the chickpeas and place in a food processor along with all of the ingredients (including the optional flavor). Pulse the mixture until it's almost smooth. If the mixture is too dry to completely get smooth add a couple of tablespoons of water, olive oil, or the juice from the chickpea can. Drizzle with olive oil or sprinkle with paprika if desired. Dip with vegetables or pita bread. Or use as a condiment spread.

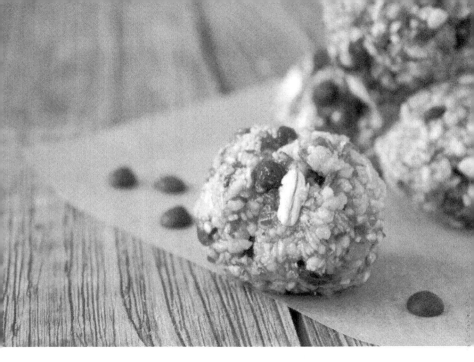

Energy Cookie Balls

Yields 15 Cookie Balls | 15 Minutes

Mix all ingredients together in a bowl (or mix together in stand mixer) until sticky and can form into a ball. Keep in refrigerator until ready to eat for best results.

Vegetarian Plan Tip:
Approved for vegetarians that eat eggs and/or dairy. Leave out Collagen Protein.

1 cup oats (optional)

1/4 cup flax meal

1/4 cup flax seeds and/or chia seeds

1/4 cup unsweetened shredded coconut

1 scoop Livingood Daily Collagen Protein

1/2 cup stevia-sweetened chocolate chips

1/4 cup goji berries

1 cup almond butter (more or less until sticky)

1/4 cup honey (can use water)

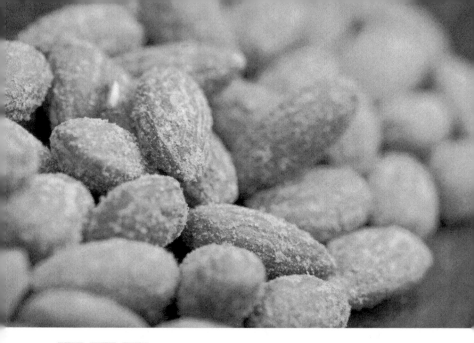

Cinnamon Baked Nuts

Yields 2 Cups | 25 Minutes - 1 Hour

2 cups raw almonds
(or any other nut)

2 tsp cinnamon

1/2 tsp sea salt

1 tbsp coconut or avocado oil

Toss all ingredients into a large bowl. Spread out on a parchment paper lined baking dish. Roast for 1 hour at 250 degrees F.

Anti-Inflammatory Plan Tip: Nuts and coconut oil are options for this plan, in moderation, if no known sensitivities.

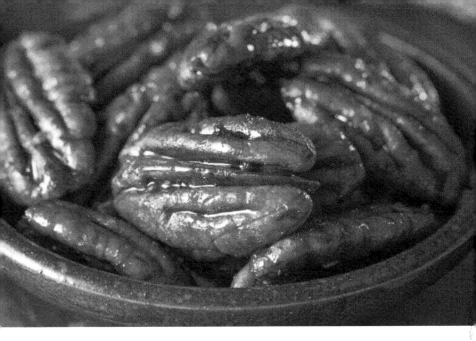

Candied Nuts

Yields 2 Cups | 20 Minutes

Toss all ingredients into a large bowl. Spread out on a parchment paper lined baking dish. Bake 350 degrees F for 15-20 minutes. Cool and enjoy!

Anti-Inflammatory Plan Tip:
Coconut oil, butter, and nuts are options for this plan, in moderation, if no known sensitivities.

Low Carb Plan Tip:
Instead of maple syrup, put all ingredients under low carb option in small pot on low heat until melted and pour over nuts before baking.

2 cups raw pecans (or any other nut)

1 tbsp coconut oil

2 tbsp yakon syrup, maple syrup, or coconut nectar

1/2 tsp sea salt

Low Carb Option:
2 tbsp butter or coconut oil

1/2 tsp vanilla extract

1 tbsp Swerve sweetner or stevia

1 tsp cinnamon

Sea salt (to taste)

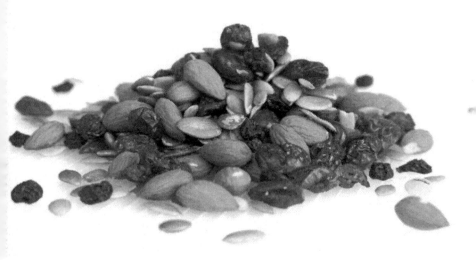

Make Your Own Trail Mix
Yields 6-7 Cups | 5 Minutes

3 cups of raw nuts of choice (almond, cashew, brazil, walnut, pecan, pistachios, hazelnut)

1 cup of raw seed of choice (pumpkin, sunflower)

1 cup stevia-sweetened chocolate chips

1/2 cup unsweetened coconut flakes

1/2 cup goji berries

1 cup dried fruit (optional - raisins, cranberries, unsweetened bananas, unsweetened mangoes, apricots, apples)

Mix all ingredients together in a large bowl or baggie and have on hand for go-to snacks.

Anti-Inflammatory Plan Tip: Nuts are an option for this plan, in moderation, if no known sensitivities. Remove chocolate chips.

Low Carb Plan Tip: Leave out the goji berries and optional dried fruit.

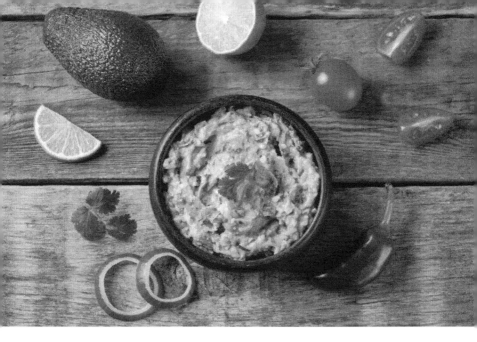

Guacamole

Yields 2 Cups | 15 Minutes

Mix avocado, lime juice, garlic, salt and pepper well until smooth consistency. Add in diced tomatoes, cilantro, and red onion and mix well. Serve with vegetables such as carrots, cucumbers, bell peppers, or celery.

Anti-Inflammatory Plan Tip: Tomatos are an option for this plan, in moderation, if no known sensitivities.

3 ripe avocados

1 juice of a lime

1 clove of garlic (minced) or garlic powder/salt

Salt and pepper (to taste)

1 roma tomato (diced)

1/4 cup cilantro (chopped)

1/8 cup red onion (finely diced)

Optional: jalapeños (diced)

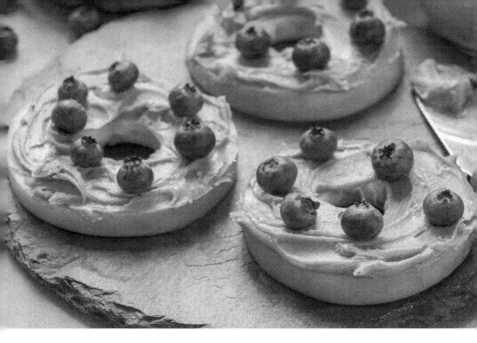

Green Apple Snacks
Serves 1 | 10 Minutes

Nut Butter Apples:
1 granny smith apple (sliced in thin slices)

Almond butter

Honey

Cinnamon

Blueberries or raisins (optional)

Apple Cinnamon Slices:
1 granny smith apple (sliced in thin slices)

Cinnamon

Swerve granular sugar

Nut Butter Apples:
Pretty simple here! Lay sliced apples on a plate and drizzle or dip apples in the almond butter. Sprinkle with whatever toppings you desire!

Apple Cinnamon Slices:
Slice the apple in thin slices. Sprinkle with cinnamon and/or Swerve "sugar". Bake at 350 degrees F for approximately 10 minutes or until soft.

Anti-Inflammatory Plan Tip:
Nut butters are an option for this plan, in moderation, if no known sensitivities.

Low Carb Plan Tip:
Be sure to use granny smith apples for a low carb plan. Also, avoid toppings like honey and raisins if doing low carb.

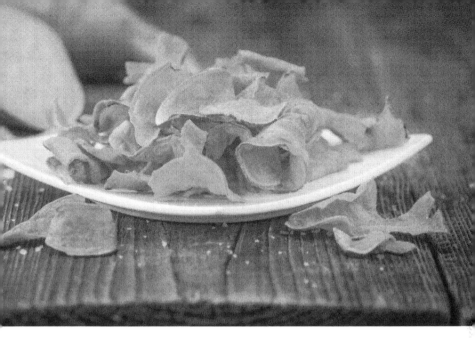

Sweet Potato Chips

Serves 1 | 10 Minutes + 2 Hours

Slice the sweet potatoes as uniformly and thin as possible. You can also use a mandoline slicer or peeler. The thinner the slice, the crisper it will be. Toss the sweet potatoes in the coconut oil until lightly coated and sprinkle with sea salt. Lay out the potatoes in a single layer on a baking sheet and bake for approximately 2 hours at 250 degrees F. Flip them half way through. Remove from oven and let rest for about 10 minutes before removing them from the pan and eating to allow them to crisp up!

Anti-Inflammatory Plan Tip:
Replace coconut oil with avocado oil, if sensitive.

2 sweet potatoes

2 tbsp coconut or avocado oil

1/4 tsp sea salt

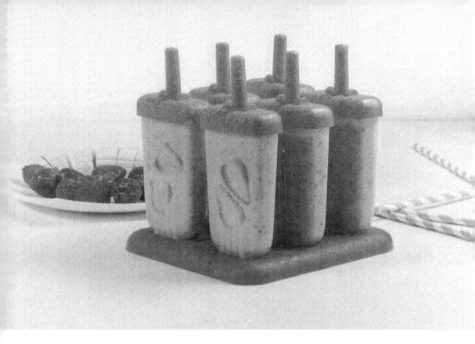

Homemade Popsicles

Yields 6 Popsicles | 15 Minutes + Freeze Time

Berry Base:
1 can coconut milk

2 tbsp maple syrup (optional)

1 tsp vanilla extract (optional)

1/2-1 scoop Livingood Daily
Collagen Protein or Greens
(optional)

Berry:
2 cups berries of choice

1/2 scoop Livingood Daily
Berry Greens powder
(optional)

1 tbsp lime juice (optional)

Fruit:
2 cups fruit of choice
(pineapple, mango, banana)

Put all ingredients in a blender and then fill popsicle molds. Store in freezer and enjoy within 6 months.

Anti-Inflammatory Plan Tip: Coconut milk are options for this plan as well as chocolate, cacao, and coffee, in moderation, if no known sensitivities.

Low Carb Plan Tip: Avoid the honey or maple syrup and use the Livingood Daily Collagen Protein.

Vegetarian Plan Tip: Use a vegetarian protein or Livingood Daily Greens in place of the Collagen Protein.

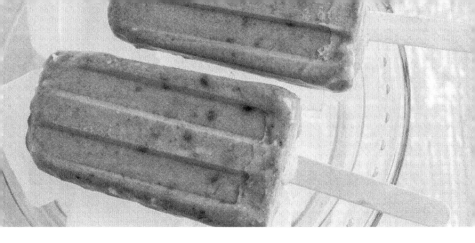

Homemade Popsicles (Continued)

Continued From Previous Page

Put all ingredients in a blender and then fill popsicle molds. Store in freezer and enjoy within 6 months.

If you do not have Livingood Daily Chocolate Collagen you can easily substitue 1-2 tbsp of cocoa powder.

Chocolate Base:
1 can coconut milk

2 tbsp honey or maple syrup (optional)

1 tsp vanilla extract (optional)

1/2-1 scoop Livingood Daily Chocolate Collagen Protein (optional)

Chocolate Crunch:
1 scoop Livingood Daily Chocolate Greens

1/4 cup stevia-sweetened chocolate chips

3 tbsp cacao nibs

Chocolate Fudgsicle:
1 scoop Livingood Daily Chocolate Greens

1/2 - 1 avocado

Pinch of salt

Chocolate Coffee:
2 cups organic coffee (cold) or 1-2 tsp instant organic coffee or espresso powder

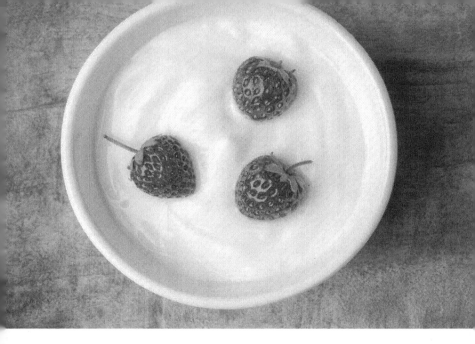

Fruit Honey-Yogurt Dip

Yields 1 Cup | 10 Minutes + Chill Time

1 cup plain, grass-fed yogurt
or full-fat greek yogurt

2 tbsp honey or **1/2** scoop
Livingood Daily Vanilla
Collagen

1 tsp cinnamon (optional)

Combine all ingredients in a bowl
until mixed well. Cover and place in
refrigerator until ready to use. Dip
your favorite fruits in this yummy dip.

Low Carb Plan Tip:
Can substitute the honey with stevia
sweetener, Livingood Daily Collagen
Proetin, or remove all together.

Vegetarian Plan Tip:
Approved for vegetarians that eat
eggs and/or dairy.

Made in the USA
Coppell, TX
01 February 2022

72788670R00114